BELOVED SON
Born with HIV

BELOVED SON

Born with HIV

by Thérèse Muamini
with Nadine Bitner

translated from the French
by Barbara Bray

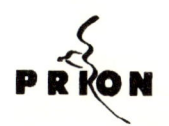

PRION

First published in France by Editions Ramsay 1995
as *Mons fils, mon amour*

First published in Great Britain by PRION
32–34 Gordon House Road,
London NW5 1LP

© Copyright Editions Ramsay 1995
English translation © Copyright Prion 1995

All rights reserved. No part of this book may be reproduced or transmitted in any form or by any means, electronic or mechanical, including photocopying and recording, or by any information storage or retrieval system, without permission in writing from the publisher and copyright holder

A catalogue record of this book can be obtained from the British Library

ISBN 1–85375–202–9 Paperback
ISBN 1–85375–205–3 Cased

Typeset in 12/14pt Baskerville by
Books Unlimited (Nottm), Mansfield NG19 7QZ
Printed and bound in Great Britain by
Biddles Ltd, Guildford & Kings Lynn

Cover image: Tony Stone Images/Phil Borges
Photograph of Thérèse & Tshakua: Patrick Bartholomew

Contents

CHAPTER ONE
My story is my son's   9

CHAPTER TWO
The terrible years   39

CHAPTER THREE
My own choice   85

CHAPTER FOUR
He's got the virus but he isn't ill   125

CHAPTER FIVE
He's my child, entrusted to me by God   161

Afterword I   183

Afterword II   189

CHAPTER ONE

My story is my son's

My story begins when Tshakua and his mother, Mme B., arrived in France. That was in 1983. I'd been here myself since 1976. I was still living with the man friend I had at the time, and I was working as a cleaner. One day I received a letter telling me they were coming and would soon be here. I was so pleased to see them: for me she'd always been like a sister. In fact, whenever I mention her, even now, I always call her "my sister". It would be nearer the truth, though, to say she was a cousin, because my village in Rwanda's made up of about twenty houses, straw huts, and we're all just one big family. An ancestor settled in the village, got married and stayed on there, the children grew up, married in their turn, and so our community has gone on ever since, living its peaceful life there in the forest near the river.

Tshakua was only a baby when Mme B. brought him over; she'd left her older children behind with her husband. Officially she was here as a tourist, but her real idea was to get away from her own country for a while: her husband wanted to have other wives and she was against it. So she came to France for a change of scene.

This polygamy business is distressing. I have very painful memories of my own childhood because of it. It wrecks people's lives, because when a man's got three wives he never treats them equally. When the father marries a second wife it means, whatever anybody may say, that he's stopped loving the first one, or at least doesn't love her as much as he used to. And she's supposed just to put up with his giving his love to someone else. The wives don't usually rebel – they haven't got the power; but they do suffer. In our house, when my mother was angry with my father she didn't take it out on him or the other wives: she turned on us children.

I can see myself now with my father when I was a very little girl. When he was eating, he liked having me at his side, either to share the meal or just to watch, in which case he would let me taste the different dishes. I loved these moments; he was a chief, and I was proud that the chief should want his daughter beside him. Sometimes it wasn't me that he called, but his son. Whenever anyone else took my place I was sick with jealousy. I regarded it as my place. In fact, he would seek me out when there was a calm atmosphere between him and my mother, but if they'd been quarrelling and he was in a bad mood – not on your life! I was a woman, and I was punished for it. On days like that my mother was harsh with us. I know it wasn't her fault: she was beside herself with jealousy. But I was unhappy too. I wasn't allowed to go where my father was, and where there were other children, and I wasn't allowed to talk to my mother either. She was angry, she rejected me – she might even give me a cuff or two if she was especially cross. The women in our society are unhappy, but nobody's interested. The men go on doing just as they please, and the women aren't supposed to say anything. All they can do to express their feelings is scold their poor children.

Maybe it was this kind of experience that made me feel I must take my life into my own hands, and in particular come to Europe. If I'd had a sheltered and happy childhood I'd probably have stayed tied to my mother's apron-strings. As it was, I left my village very early on. I remember making up my mind I'd never suffer as the other women in my country did. I'd only live with a man who believed in monogamy.

My sister wasn't happy either.

When she arrived in Paris Tshakua was eight months old. He was born in July 1982. I went to meet them at the airport, and immediately loved the baby. He was beautiful, with a very light skin, big hands and feet. He never cried. A real darling.

We spent the day together so glad to be re-united. We'd always been very close, and were both looking forward to our time together.

And then all of a sudden, during the night, she started moaning.

"I've got a terrible headache!"

She had a temperature. I'd given her my bed

and was sleeping on the floor. The next thing I knew, she'd fallen out of bed and was having some kind of fit. I'd never seen anything so frightening; I didn't know what was happening. Then she came to and asked me to give her the baby to feed.

The next morning we called a doctor and he prescribed some sedatives. As he left, he handed me a card and said:

"If she isn't better soon, bring her here."

It was the hospital for tropical diseases, and as her temperature didn't go down my friend and I took her in. They did all sorts of examinations and tests, then told us they needed to do a scan. They found she had a brain tumour. I began to feel terribly worried and wondered what we were going to do.

She'd arrived here on the Saturday, been taken ill the same night, was still unwell on the Sunday, and by Monday she was in hospital – and all without any papers or social security! As far as the social security were concerned it was all right: they had no choice but to look after her. The trouble was, I had to go out to work, and I couldn't leave a baby of eight months alone at home. We saw some social workers to find out what they could do, and they soon solved the problem, putting him in a crèche.

At least that worry was taken care of, but of course the baby was now alone among strangers. What was more, he was used to being breast-fed: he'd never even seen a bottle. The people in the crèche did all they could to get him used to their ways, but it was no good: the little boy who'd been so placid and cheerful when he arrived now cried all day and all night.

With the baby in the crèche and the mother in hospital, I just went back and forth between them and my work. Hospital, crèche, work...Work, crèche, hospital... My sister couldn't speak a word of French, so I had to be there to translate everything, even when they just asked her her name. As for the baby, he wouldn't let anyone come near him. I was worried, tired and depressed, and became very thin.

The doctors decided to remove the mother's tumour. The operation went well and she came out of hospital. But meanwhile they'd done some tests and found something wrong. They sent for me and my friend and told us the effects of the tumour might be lasting: my sister might never get back to normal after such a serious operation. And there was also something wrong with her blood.

"What?" we asked.

"We don't know yet. We'll have to wait for the results of further tests. But we know already that it's serious."

Later on they told us it was a virus. What kind of virus?

"The AIDS virus."

Whenever people use words I don't understand and no one explains them, I always think they must mean something terrible. I didn't know what the words meant then, but I was so frightened I cried. I couldn't stop! It was a bolt from the blue. How ill was she? How were we going to manage?

I'd never heard the word AIDS before, I didn't even know there was such an illness. In 1983 people didn't talk about it as they do now.

Already my sister struck me as very changed. Back in Rwanda she'd been warm-hearted and lively, always singing and dancing. But here she was completely different – depressed, and weeping all the time. They'd shaved off so much of her hair for the operation they advised us to buy her a wig. Her baby had had to be weaned, and she couldn't even see him. She was too tired for him to be brought home from the crèche: anyone would be after such a serious operation.

There was no question of my going and taking the baby out of the crèche myself. I had too much else to do. The operation had been very expensive, and someone had to go to the hospital to apply for help in paying for it. She wasn't strong enough, so my friend and I had to go and fill in all the forms.

Then, because they'd found out that the mother had the virus, they took the baby into hospital for tests. They sent for me again.

"The baby has something wrong with it. And it may turn out to be serious."

"What is it?"

"The virus."

I couldn't believe it.

"But that's impossible! He seems fine, he's not sick!"

They said there was no doubt about it: they'd found the virus in his blood. All the way home I could only stare at the ground as I went along, wondering how I was going to deal with the situation.

*

Tshakua was still in the crèche. At first he wouldn't eat; he didn't like anything they offered him. Then he settled down a bit. Sometimes one of the staff would prepare his bottle and I would give it to him. They gave him little jars of factory-made baby food, carrot purée or whatever, and he began to get used to it. And so the days went by.

At the time my sister arrived in France, my friend and I weren't getting on with one another any more, and were on the point of splitting up.

I'd met him in France in 1979. He was in the army, and had come here on a course. But now his studies were finished and he wanted to go back home. He thought I'd be going with him, but I refused.

"No, I don't want to go back. Husbands in our country like women too much, and once you're back again you'll be just like the rest. I'm staying. I want to live in Europe now. What would I do back home? Here I have a job and earn my own living. There it's the man who works – I'd have to stay at home and I'd be so miserable. I won't go back with you."

So I stayed on, and kept his son Pierre with me. He said he'd rather stay in France with me than go back to Rwanda, so his father let him. Pierre was only five or six years old when he came to France: my friend had brought all his four children here with him from Rwanda. As a matter of fact they weren't his – they were his sister's children really. Anyway he brought them over, then all except Pierre went back again. And as I was living with his father then, Pierre became my own child. He's grown-up now, eighteen, but I brought him up and he looks on me as his mother: he can't remember anything about the time before he lived with me. He's left home now, though. He's found a French girlfriend and they're living together.

Pierre's father wasn't my first man friend. I came to France in 1976 with another fellow-countryman, a doctor who lived in France but had come to Rwanda on vacation. He was very fond of me, and I of him. He was very kind, and willing to do anything I wanted: get me a house in Rwanda, or take me with him to France if I preferred. I decided to go to France with him: he was very good to me, and I hadn't got anything to my name in Rwanda, not even a job. So he paid my fare – I couldn't have afforded it myself – and we came to France together.

Whenever he came back to Rwanda on holiday, people used to treat him as a big boss. He'd won a scholarship to go and study in France, and he brought his wife and one of their children with him. Their other six children were all born here. They lived in Bordeaux. After he'd finished his studies and got his degree, he went back to Rwanda with his wife and the three youngest children, leaving the older ones in France – they had grants to help cover the cost of their education. Back in Rwanda, their father set up as a doctor in the capital. He was already well-known, he had European qualifications, and it wasn't long before he was making plenty of money. Then he started leading a life of luxury, with a big house and working in a big hospital as well as being a private consultant. He was growing really rich. But he wasn't getting on with his wife any more. In Europe they'd lived like Europeans, but as soon as the husband got back to his own country he'd started going out and coming home late. She hadn't studied medicine herself, but she'd been to the university. She knew she could earn a good living on her own, and so she asked for a divorce

It was when they split up that he and I began to see a lot of one another. But it wasn't official; I wasn't in love with him yet. Then he decided he wanted to be a specialist or a professor, and as all his studies had been done in Europe and some of his children were still there, he applied for another grant. When he got it he went back to Bordeaux, and we only saw him in Rwanda in the holidays. Meanwhile his divorce had gone through, so we didn't have to hide any more when he came. Then, after his month's vacation was up, he was due to go back to Bordeaux. So when he asked me to choose between coming to Europe or having a house in Rwanda where he could stay when he came over on holiday, I chose Europe.

After a while we parted. But as I liked it in France, I stayed.

When my sister came here I'd just met somebody else, Kasongo. Kasongo and I adopted Tshakua together. He accepted Tshakua, and he accepted my sister too. But there was a problem: we didn't have anywhere to live. Kasongo lived in a hostel, and I was staying with friends. How were we going to keep the mother and baby with us? She wanted her baby; she cried for it. I went to the crèche and asked what I could do.

"We can't let you have the baby unless you've got somewhere to live." they said. "And if you do find a place, we'll have to come and see if it's suitable."

By this time my sister had been in Paris for a year. She was living with me and beginning to feel better. The baby was growing and had started to walk. We used to go to see him in the crèche, and sometimes I even went and brought him home for the weekend. And then suddenly she fell ill again. Very ill. She had to go into hospital. From one day to the next she couldn't walk or talk or do anything for herself. Her mouth was all twisted; she couldn't keep it straight.

I knew some of the professors at the hospital and made an appointment to see them.

"What's wrong with her, professor?" I asked.

"We don't know. We'll have to see. It's the virus."

Then the baby had to go into hospital too. They wanted to keep him under observation, do some tests, watch how he got on, because there'd been some kind of warning signal. His mother could only communicate by signs now. She was in one room and the little boy was in another. She gestured that she wanted to see him, so I went and fetched him. Her mouth was still twisted and she couldn't walk, but she wanted to take care of her baby. Looking at the two of them, I began to weep.

Then the baby came out of hospital and went back to the crèche.

The mother was in hospital for four or five months that time. I used to go and see her, and I used to go and see the baby too. First one and then the other. I didn't hide the truth from Kasongo.

"The doctors say they don't know yet how her case will turn out," I told him. "But the disease has taken hold, and there isn't much hope."

What was I to do? I didn't want to leave the baby in the crèche, and had made up my mind to have him to live with me. But how could I do that without a proper place to take him to? We'd been hunting desperately for a flat to rent, but we couldn't find one. Then one day we heard about a place out at Saint-Denis that was available on hire-purchase, and we went to see it. It was very comfortable, with several bedrooms, a living-dining room, kitchen, bathroom and plenty of space. A real home. They told us the price, we went to see the banks, and Kasongo's bank agreed to lend us the money. Then the social worker in charge of Tshakua at the crèche got in touch with a social worker in Saint-Denis, and between them they arranged for us to have Tshakua with us.

It was Kasongo who went to collect him. I was working all day, and his hours were more convenient. Tshakua's mother was out of hospital by then, and we had her to live with us – Kasongo, Tshakua, me and Pierre. We gave my sister a room of her own to share with her little boy.

Everything seemed to be working out. The mother was better. She was up and about; she could even do some cooking and help look after the baby. We were glad to have him with us, we all got on very well together, life was happy and cheerful.

The mother still had to go to the hospital regularly. We only had to take the little boy in from time to time. And then one evening when I came home from work, she wasn't there.

"What's the matter?"

They told me she'd felt unwell and gone to the hospital. I didn't worry too much because I knew her: the slightest thing wrong and off she'd rush. It was a Saturday, and late. So I decided I'd wait and go and see her in the morning.

When I arrived, she was lying down on the bed, not moving.

"What's wrong?" I asked.

"My head! It hurts!"

"I've brought you something to eat," I said. "You must eat to get your strength back."

She'd never got used to the insipid food you get in France – salads and plain grilled meat. She didn't like it and and used to leave everything, even the bread. And when I went to see her she'd give it all to me.

"Here, take it for the children," she'd say. "I can't eat it."

In our country we use lots of seasoning and tomatoes in our cooking. So whenever she had to go into hospital I used to bring in some of our own sort of food for her straight away. But that morning, when I tried to give it to her, she wouldn't take it.

"No, I can't eat anything."

I pressed her.

"You ought to try!"

But she wouldn't.

"Just leave it here, and if I get hungry, I'll eat it."

I stayed with her for a while and tried to cheer her up.

"Don't worry, it won't last long! You've had much worse before. It'll soon go."

She shook her head slowly.

"It's serious this time. I know."

I didn't believe this, and tried to reason with her.

"No, it's not serious!" I said. "You're always scared and worrying yourself unnecessarily"

I knew her quite well. She was younger than I was and I'd often seen her take a pessimistic view of things.

"You're going to get better!" I told her. "You shouldn't always think the worst."

"No," she answered. "This time I know I won't get over it."

Before my sister went into hospital, she'd made friends with another out-patient, a woman who was from Rwanda too. When she became seriously ill and paralysed down one side, this woman had been in a bed nearby. My sister had grown very fond of her. But this other woman had recently died which depressed and greatly affected my sister.

"She died, didn't she? And she was just as young as I am!"

I tried to convince her their two cases were quite different. I did my best to take her mind off the subject of death. But she wouldn't listen. It was getting late. I stood up to go.

"I have to go. I have to see to the children."

"Take good care of Tshakua. If anything ever happens to me, I don't want you to abandon him. Promise me you'll never leave him."

"I promise," I said. "But I know nothing's going to happen to you."

But she was still very sad.

"There's no point in coming to see me," she said. "Just phone. No, don't phone – you're too busy. And there's no need for you to come back this evening. Stay with the children and look after Tshakua."

When I got home, Tshakua was there with Kasongo and Pierre. As soon as he saw me, Tshakua rushed up to me calling out "Mummy, Mummy!"

He'd got into the habit of calling me that because he'd seen so much of me when he was a baby, in the crèche. He called his mother "Auntie". In his eyes I was already his mother.

I have a child of my own, one I brought into the world myself. He's twenty-three years old now and lives in Rwanda. I couldn't bring him with me when I came to France with the doctor, and later on, when I wanted to have him with me, he didn't want to come. He was born when I was seventeen or eighteen, and I had malaria when I was expecting him. I saw the doctor and he prescribed some medicine, but I was careless and didn't take it regularly. So when the baby was born we both had malaria. He had a fever and needed care. I breast-fed him, but it was my mother who really looked after him. She was better at it than I was. I was even a bit jealous.

My mother had never had a son herself. But she was still young, and glad to inherit that fine little boy from me. She came to think of him as her own, as is often the way in our country. So much so that when I came to France she said:

"He's my child and I don't want to lose him."

But I love him too, and when I go back to Rwanda I'm always happy to see him. I love him, but not in the way I love Tshakua. Tshakua is my real child, because I brought him up.

They kept my sister on in the hospital over the Saturday and Sunday. I phoned up three times a day: in the morning when I got to work, at the midday break, and in the evening before I went home. When I phoned up on the Monday they told me her condition was stable. The same on the Tuesday. I called up again on the Wednesday.

"I'm inquiring about Mme B."

"Are you a friend of hers?"

Then they said she wasn't there.

"But she was there before!"

"Yes, but she's been transferred."

I was getting uneasy.

"Has anything happened to her?"

"We can't tell you anything over the phone. Come in and we'll explain."

I hadn't started work yet, so I told the woman in charge I couldn't do anything that morning – I had to go to the hospital.

When I got there I went up to the room where I'd seen her last, anyway. The person I'd spoken to on the phone might have made a mistake. I didn't want to think why my sister might have been transferred to another department.

I found her bed empty but I still didn't panic, I just asked where I had to go to see her.

"In emergency," they said. "In intensive care."

So I went there. I was beginning to wonder what it all meant.

"I want to see Mme B."

"Sorry – you can't."

"Why?"

"You'll have to wait and see the doctor."

I waited. I didn't jump to any conclusions: she'd had much worse before. I told myself this was nothing more. A moment later I saw her doctor, a woman – but she walked straight past me without a word or a look. This struck me as strange: she usually said hello and talked to me for a while. But I thought she must just be in a hurry, and I went on waiting. Finally the doctor came out of the ward and walked over to where I was.

"Be brave!" she said.

"What do you mean, 'brave'"?

"It's finished," she said. "Her life is over."

I don't think I'd ever had such a shock in all my life. I was completely unprepared for it. Although my sister spoke despairingly on Saturday, I hadn't really listened to her. Then she'd been moved to another ward, and her doctor had hurried past me without speaking. And still I'd clung to my illusions.

Everything had been going so well. Everyone at home had been happy as recently as Friday evening... and now this! Of course I'd known it was serious, very serious – that virus she had in her blood: the doctor hadn't concealed it from us. But she had been so well. She could walk, she was leading a normal life, she was doing some cooking – there'd been no reason to think she was going to die. When she was paralysed and her mouth was all twisted to one side, then I thought about it. But after that she'd got back to normal again – we used to go out together, do the shopping, laugh and have fun together like a couple of kids. Then all of a sudden she was ill – and now dead. I couldn't take it in.

I'd thought she was cured and out of danger, but that was only how it looked. In fact she still had that horrible virus in her blood.

"She was still seriously ill," the doctor said.

I went in and saw her lying there on the bed. But I hadn't the strength to come away again. I just crawled about on the floor of that hospital room like a wounded animal, and just lay there. I couldn't get over the shock. I knew people were looking at me, and I'd have liked to get up, but I couldn't. It had all happened too quickly.

Finally I dragged myself to the phone and called Kasongo. It calmed me down a bit to hear his voice.

"Wait there, I'm coming."

So I sat there on the floor, stunned and unable to move. Kasongo came and took me home, then went to collect the baby from the crèche. He was the one who took him there every morning and brought him home every evening. Tshakua was still very young then: he was born in 1982 and his mother died in 1985.

But he'd already acquired a habit that's made it difficult to bring him up properly. Whenever he's scolded he gets upset: he withdraws into himself and is so miserable you can't help going and trying to comfort him.

When I saw him that day I started to cry. I still couldn't believe his mother was dead: it wasn't possible, it wasn't true. All my memories flooded back. I kept saying, "But why? We bought this flat so that we could be happy, and now the happiness is gone!" I took the little boy in my arms and couldn't stop crying.

I tried to pull myself together. "Come on! I must try to forget and think only of the child. His mother's gone, and now I'm the only mother he's got. I must look after him as if he were my own. Better than if he were my own."

And I have given him all that anyone could. I

didn't even know, then, that I was capable of doing what I've done. I'd left my own child, the one I actually bore, back in Rwanda with my mother. But for Tshakua I found all the love that was in me. I've grown fonder of him than of my own child, than of anyone else in the world, and I've fought for him every day of my life from that day to this.

Kasongo and I went to see the judge and he gave us custody. It took some time because we had to produce all sorts of documents. Then we had to go through a long process to get the family allowance people to recognise the situation. We waited and waited for them to complete the file, but in the end it was all right. And so we all lived together – Tshakua, my husband and I – and Tshakua became my son.

He's not adopted – he really is my son. It's the same as when a man and a woman love each other, really love each other. If one day they decide to get married officially it's a mere formality, a gesture to the State. They say to each other: "We love each other, so we'll regularise our situation." And why not? But for my part, if I ask myself "What do I feel, deep down?" – well, whether I've been before the judge or not, Tshakua is my child. If it had all happened back in my own country we wouldn't even have had to go through any legal hoops. Out there, if the father or mother dies, the child is looked after by anyone who's able to do so – a sister, say, or an aunt. It isn't the same back there as it is in France, where most families have only one or two children! We have lots of them. One family may have ten, twenty children, and there isn't always enough food to go round. So even if the mother of three or four children is still alive, her girlfriend or sister will take on one of them if she's in a better position to care for it.

If I were the mother I'd go and suckle the baby, but I'd leave it with my friend or sister, and she'd look after it until it's grown up. It's the custom.

I have kept this way of looking at things, and I acted as I would have done back home. And that's why I know, deep down, that Tshakua really is my child. And no one can ever take him away from me The judge handed him over to us when his mother died, and since then he's been my responsibility for life.

There's another thing. When you're given custody of a child the social workers make enquiries to ensure he's being properly looked after. To find out whether to leave him with you or take him away. But they don't do that with me any more: he's happy and healthy and everyone is pleased with me. People tell me I ought to go back to the judge now with all my family and get permanent custody, but I don't think it's necessary. I know very well Tshakua's mine. What I think is, if they do give me permanent custody it won't change anything because he's already mine; and even if they don't, he'll still be mine anyway. So I don't bother about it. I don't write, and I don't go and see the judge. I've been sure he's my child ever since the doctor told me his mother had something serious the matter with her and it wasn't certain she'd live.

Tshakua was still only eight months old, and I knew he was going to be mine. I'd made up my mind.

The social workers have often talked to me about it.

"We used to make regular inquiries to find out how you were looking after him. But that stage is over," they say. "What you have to do now is make up your mind and go to see the judge, before witnesses, and then you'll be given permanent custody."

But to tell you the truth I don't feel like it. Perhaps I'm being careless. But I won't go.

So I went on living with my friend Kasongo, Tshakua and Pierre. We were happy together. And we took good care of Tshakua.

When he first got ill he was given AZT[†] in liquid form. The doctor said he must take it at regular intervals, which meant we had to wake him up at midnight. At first we were so scared of missing the right time we used to set the alarm for twelve o'clock sharp. When we went to stay with friends he couldn't be left to sleep with the other children: we had to have him in with us so we could give him his medicine on the stroke of midnight.

The number of times he had to stay away from school was another problem. In the early years he was always ill with a temperature or ear-ache or swollen glands. And if the hospital tests showed

---

[†] AZT is the drug zivodudine, the earliest to obtain some positive results in the treatment of HIV patients. It is now more commonly used in combination with newer drugs.

anything unusual the doctors would keep him in for a week or so until he was better. But we had to explain to the school why he'd been away, so we were always trying to find new excuses. We couldn't tell the truth; we were forced to lie. And the school was always asking me for his health record – the little book every child has containing his vaccination record, so that he gets his jabs at the proper intervals. But I knew it would be very dangerous for him to be vaccinated: it had to be avoided at all costs. But of course I couldn't say that. I had to tell them I'd lost the book, or something.

Having to tell lies all the time made life very complicated. If friends invited us to go and see them we had to take a syringe with us and measure Tshakua's medicine out in secret. And we used to keep our luggage and my handbag with us all the time in case someone should go through our things and find a whole chemist's shop of drugs.

We lived like that for some time. And then one day my friend Kasongo left me.

All the ordeals I'd been through had left me depressed: Tshakua's mother's death, Tshakua's illness, and so on. I suffered from spasms because I was so unhappy, and Kasongo couldn't cheer me up. I had some out-patient treatment. I saw some psychologists. But they only said I must try to help myself. So, as my mother wasn't well, I decided to go back home for a while to see her and to try and sort myself out. My mother died while I was out there, and I fell ill again, worse than before. Then, when I got back to France, Kasongo told me he was leaving me. Just like that, without any explanation.

"But why?"

"Just because."

I'd left Tshakua with Kasongo when I went away: I couldn't take him with me because he had to go to the hospital once a fortnight. But even when I was in France it was Kasongo who'd looked after him most of the time. I worked hard as a cleaner in Paris and didn't finish till nine in the evening. It was ten by the time I got home. In the morning too, Kasongo started work later than I did. I began at seven, but he had time to get Tshakua ready for school, and then, as he had the car, he used to drive him there. In the afternoon Kasongo used to finish work at four o'clock, buy something at the baker's for Tshakua's tea, and at half-past four collect him from school. Tshakua was really more attached to Kasongo than he was to me, because he saw more of him. Kasongo was always there, washing and dressing him in the morning and giving him his breakfast, just like a mother. And on the days when Tshakua had to go to the hospital, Kasongo dropped him there on his way to work and went and fetched him home later on.

When Kasongo told me he was leaving, I wondered how on earth I was going to solve all my problems. He'd met another woman. I was quite willing to see his point of view, but how was I going to manage? I'd lost my job when I returned to Rwanda, and now I'd have to try to find another.

As for the flat we'd started to buy, Kasongo had stopped paying the monthly instalments when he met his new girlfriend. I didn't know about this until the owners sent in the bailiffs, sold the flat to someone else, and threw us out. Kasongo just packed his bags and left. But what was I to do, with no job, nowhere to live, and three children to look after, one of them ill?

I say three children because by now I had another one on my hands, Sango, my brother's son. When I was in Rwanda to see my mother, my brother asked me to take his son back to France with me. He himself would come and join us soon. Sango was three years old when he came here, and the new life wasn't easy for him. He didn't speak a word of French, and had to spend a lot of time with Tshakua, who didn't speak anything else. And at first Sango ate next to nothing: he wasn't used to seeing so much food. My brother did come to France some time later, but I looked after Sango from 1988 till 1990, while his father looked for work and somewhere to live. When he found a place his wife came over too, and then he took Sango back again.

So, when Kasongo left, I went to see the social worker.

"All I can do," she said, "is take the children away and place them with the Department of Health and Social Services."

"That's the last thing I'd agree to," I told her. "Just leave my Tshakua alone. I saw how unhappy he was in the crèche. Do you think I'd let him be sent back there now, after he's been with me? No, not for anything in the world!"

I decided to try to manage on my own. How I had to struggle! I couldn't even get family allowance for the children; all I had was my unemployment pay. It wasn't much, and the social worker didn't help.

"There's nothing I can do for you if you won't give in!" she used to say. "Seeing you haven't got a job or anywhere to live, I'm supposed to take the children away from you."

"I know that," I'd told her. "But I won't let you."

I'd got through the first ordeal – the death of Tshakua's mother. And then through Tshakua's own illness. Now I had to get over the next hurdle, with three children to provide for. And I still had to go on hiding the medicine! If by any chance anyone agreed to put us up for a few days, that was always a problem. It's easy enough if you're in your own place, but what are you to do when you're staying with a friend? How can you give the child his medicine without her seeing?

At that time Tshakua was still taking AZT, and I had to measure it out with a syringe. It was easy enough at night, when I had him sleeping with me, but what was I to do during the day? I used to keep the phials and syringes ready in my pocket or my bag. Then, when I knew no one could see, I'd take them out and call him over.

"Come along, darling, open wide! There! All over!"

Where did we live? Three days here, a week

there, a couple of days somewhere else.

At last I found some work. Again as a cleaner. "Thank you, God!" I thought, and started looking for a hotel. I found one in the middle of Saint-Denis. It cost a hundred francs a day. A hundred francs – but you weren't allowed to do any cooking in your room. As a cleaner I earned three thousand francs a month: fifteen hundred in the mornings and fifteen hundred in the evenings, and it all went on paying for the hotel. But I'd made up my mind. I wasn't going to let them take Tshakua away from me.

I might have agreed to part with Pierre. There was nothing the matter with him. But when it came to Tshakua – I wouldn't even consider it. So I went and lived in that hotel with the children. Everything was a struggle. Life was horribly difficult. All the money I earned went on paying the hotel bill, and the social worker wouldn't do anything for me.

"I can't help you if you won't let the Department of Health and Social Services take charge of the children," she said.

One day I even stole for my children. What an awful thing to do! But it was so difficult to give them enough to eat.

They ate in the school canteen at midday; I usually skipped lunch, myself. But Wednesday was a holiday and there was no canteen. One Wednesay when I hadn't any money left and was at my wits' end, I went into a supermarket and took a salami sausage and hid it under my coat. And then I took some ham. And all the time I was thinking, "So long as the children get something to eat today that's all that matters."

Unfortunately there was a camera, and it had spotted me. The shop had proof against me, and as I was going out they took me aside.

"Come this way, please," they said.

I tried to explain.

"I'm sorry... I don't earn much... I've got children, and we all live in a hotel... I haven't any more money left, and this was the only way I could think of to get them something to eat."

"You haven't any more money? Empty your handbag!"

I turned my handbag upside down, and nothing at all fell out. I hadn't a penny!

"You haven't got enough to pay for all you've taken."

"I haven't got anything! Take me to the police station if you want to – I'll just tell them the truth. And the truth is, it was the only thing I could do. When I've paid the hotel bills – look, here are the receipts! A hundred francs a day! – I've spent every penny I earn."

"That's all very well," they said, "but what are we supposed to do? You stole, so you'll have to pay."

But finally they relented.

"Look, what we'll do is this: we'll photocopy your ID papers and we'll keep them on our files. And if you ever steal anything again we'll call the police, and then you can explain yourself in court!"

In court! I was so ashamed. I went away and never stole again.

CHAPTER TWO

The terrible years

For ten years I suffered.

From the time he was eight months old until he was eleven, I had a lot of pain and many disappointments. I often cried, everything was difficult. Life is hard. And these social workers, who kept on telling me they couldn't do anything for me because I wouldn't let them take the children away.

They didn't even do the things they could have done. I don't know why.

Of all my memories the one that hurts me most to think of now is something that happened often. Very often.

After they repossessed the flat a girlfriend of mine called Sylvie took us in. I'd just got back from Rwanda and was out of work, so looking for a job was my most urgent problem. Then when I found something it was in some offices in Paris, and the cleaners had to get in very early in the morning, before the people who worked there. But Sylvie lived, as we used to, out at Saint-Denis. So I had to get up at four in the morning to catch the train in to Paris, leaving Pierre to look after his brothers.

But once a fortnight Tshakua had to be taken to the hospital, and on those days I just had to get him ready and take him with me at four in the morning. He was only about six years old at the time and very delicate; I had to muffle him up against the cold in the winter. The people at my new job didn't know me yet, and wouldn't have understood if I'd asked to take the morning off once a fortnight. So while I cleaned my offices I used to sit the poor little thing down somewhere with a box of crayons, to amuse himself as best he could. Sometimes he'd fall asleep waiting for me. Then when I'd finished work I'd take him to the hospital. And I still can't help crying, even today, to think that if I'd known I could have had an ambulance call for him at home. An ambulance service was provided, and we could have made use of it. But no one told me about it. No one. And how was I supposed to guess? So it was my little boy who had to suffer, trailing about in trains, hanging around in offices in the dark and the cold, when all the time he could have been driven straight to the hospital and sat there quietly in the warm!

Sylvie, whose place we were living in for a while, was a Rwandan woman who went to the same church as I did. When I'd come home and found the flat shut up, with the bailiff's seals on the door, I'd gone to the minister for help. He knew Sylvie had just lost her husband and had some room to spare, so he asked her to take us in temporarily. She couldn't refuse.

I slept in her living room. I kept Tshakua's medicine on me all the time so she shouldn't notice anything, but I was always afraid she might find out. Then one day she told me we'd have to leave. She gave plenty of reasons. She was a widow, and not very well off as she didn't work. There were lots of old people in her building, and my children were young and rowdy. They made a noise, they'd broken a window and so on, and she was afraid of being turned out of her flat. Her husband had just died, her own papers weren't in order – what if she too found herself in the street? She wanted to be friendly and helpful, but she just couldn't take so many risks.

I tried to make her change her mind.

"Please!" I begged. "I do my best not to be in your way! I even sleep on the floor! But that doesn't matter – all I ask is for you to go on helping me till I find somewhere to live."

But she refused. If I'd been on my own she wouldn't have minded how long I stayed, but the children were too much for her. I implored. I even offered to pay the rent. But she still refused.

"I don't want any money – I put you up for nothing because it was an emergency. Maybe I could have taken something if it was a permanent arrangement. But I can't go on. I haven't got anything against you personally – you behave properly and do your share in the house – but I can't stand having the children here any longer."

I wept, and tried to make her see what a desperate situation I was in.

"At least give me one more chance to find somewhere to live."

So finally she agreed. I searched everywhere, asked everyone, was always on the watch. Then one day, when I was talking to a man I knew by sight because he went to my church, he said:

"You've got a job, and papers, and children to support. I'll find an empty house, somewhere quiet and out of the way, and draw you up a false lease. Then you give me some money, I'll force the door open, and you can go and live there. With a bit of luck no one will notice, and if by any chance the town hall or the owner starts asking questions, you just say, 'Someone offered me a lease, and that's all I know about it.' Even if that did happen I doubt if they'd turn you out, because of the children."

At first I liked the idea. "Why not?" I thought, and agreed to his suggestion. But after a while I said to myself, "It's too risky. If I put my name to a forged lease and am found out, they might take the children away from me and give them to the Social Services."

So when I saw the gentleman at church I told him I'd changed my mind.

Every Sunday Sylvie wanted to know how we were getting on.

"What news from the man who's supposed to be finding you a house?" she asked.

"I've told him it's off. I don't want to get on the wrong side of the law. I don't fancy the idea of forcing the door of a place when you don't know if the owner's alive or dead, or whether he's got a family."

Sylvie was furious.

"That's it!" she said. "This thing has got to be settled now. I want you to leave today."

"But where am I supposed to go?" I cried.

"I think you're lying to me!" she said. "You tell me you're doing all you can and asking everyone. You say you can't even find a hotel. But it's not true! You tell me someone's going to break into a house so that you can go and live there, and now you say that's off! You say the first thing that comes into your head, and I think it's all lies. So today you and I are going to do the rounds of the hotels together!"

I said I preferred to look in Saint-Denis because that was where the children's schools were. She agreed, and off we went. We must have gone to every hotel in Saint-Denis. And at every one I insisted on telling them the truth. That I had three children. They all refused to have me.

"We don't have people staying here by the month," they'd say. "And anyway it's not suitable for children."

Some said it would have been all right if I'd been on my own, or just with a man. But with the children... No, what I needed was a flat, not a room.

All the time I was praying inside my head:

"Lord, you must help me."

Before I'd set out with Sylvie I'd been to see the social worker again. She'd said the only thing for me to do was have the children taken into care until I found somewhere for us all to live. That was the sensible way to tackle the problem.

But I refused. My brother's wife still hadn't arrived, and I'd promised to look after Sango until she did. But my main reason was Tshakua. My brother could have had Sango himself if the worst came to the worst, and Pierre was probably old enough now not to come to any harm with the social services. But Tshakua – I loved him too much for that. I needed to look after him, to see he took his medicine, to watch over what he ate. I couldn't possibly give him up.

Well, Sylvie and I had been trudging round for hours, and I was explaining my situation to yet another hotel manager.

"I've got three children and nowhere to live. I'm looking for a room where the children and I can stay until I find a flat."

And this time the hotel manager didn't say no.

"Yes," he answered. "I have got a room. But there are problems."

"What problems?"

"We don't let rooms by the month – only by the day. But as you've nowhere to go... I adopted a little black girl myself, so I feel for you and would like to help you out. But only until you find somewhere permanent."

He told me his conditions. I couldn't stay in the room during the day. I couldn't do any cooking. And I had to pay a hundred francs a day or seven hundred a week.

"I'll do whatever I have to do," I thought. "I'll even pay a hundred francs a day for a hotel if I must."

I couldn't stay in the room during the day because someone came round to check from time to time, and the manager would be fined if the inspector found me. It was one of those places people go to just to make love, and you weren't allowed to have children there. I realised it was going to be difficult, but there was no alternative.

The hotel keeper and the chambermaid took us up to see the room. How wonderful! It had a little refrigerator, a little television set, and a large bed. The man showed us where we had to go to have a bath, and told us the lavatory was on the landing.

I was so relieved to have found somewhere.

I thanked my friend Sylvie for her hospitality, but deep down I was angry with her. She knew very well I didn't mean to stay on indefinitely – all I'd needed was time to solve my problem.

We went back to her place, and I packed my things and waited for the children. When they came home from school I took them to the hotel and left them there while I went to work, warning them not to make any noise. I didn't like having to leave them: I didn't know what they'd do about supper, all on their own. When I finished work and got back to the hotel I found them watching the little television. I hadn't had time before to tell them what was happening, so I told them then. Pierre was a big boy now – he was born in 1974 and this was 1989 – and he already looked after the other two like an elder brother. I explained the situation to him.

"I have to go out to work, and all I earn will go on paying for the hotel. You'll have to take my place. You're the man of the family now. You must take care of your brothers and give them their meals and so on, because I'm going to have to leave for work very early in the morning."

I can hardly bear to think of our life in that hotel. It was horrible. And yet it was a nice place, light and very clean. From the window you could see a patio with flowers in it. But it was a bad time for us.

All that came out of the tap in the morning was a tiny trickle of water. When I held my finger under it, it was cold.

"Let it run until it gets hot," I told Pierre. "If it ever does. Then mix it up with Nesquik and powdered milk, and give it to the boys with some bread and butter. If the water stays cold, too bad. You must get something inside you."

And every morning after I'd left he used to get up and dress, then wash and dress Sango and Tshakua and give them their breakfast.

Luckily there was a chambermaid in the hotel who was very kind. She was a great help to me. On the very first day, when we went up to see the room, she'd said:

"I know what it's like for you, My husband left me with three children, no job and nowhere to live. It was awful. Fortunately some people were prepared to help me. So if ever you need anything, don't hesitate to ask me and I'll give you a hand."

"There is one thing," I said. "It's about getting the children off in the morning. Tshakua's school is quite near and he can get there on his own. Pierre too. But he has to set out too early to drop Sango at nursery school."

"Don't worry," she said. "I've got a car." (She was white.) "I'll pick Sango up every morning and take him to school before I do your room."

I accepted her offer with great relief. But I still had a problem: the boys' meals, especially in the evening and at the weekend. They could manage breakfast somehow on their own, even with only cold water. In the middle of the day they had lunch in the school canteen. And I gave them biscuits or some other snack for their tea. But when I got back from work in the evening I'd find them all sitting there looking very downcast.

"We're hungry, Mum!" they'd say.

Then, when I turned the tap on:

"It's cold!" they'd shout.

It made me weep! I didn't mind spending every penny I earned. That's what you went to work for – to provide for your family. But the children must have a proper meal in the evening! And they had to have something to eat on Wednesdays, Saturdays and Sundays!

Buying the food was no problem, but I had to find somewhere to cook it. I was still too angry with Sylvie to set foot in her place. So I tried to think of other people who might let me use their kitchen. I told Emilie, a fellow-countrywoman who went to the same church as I did, about the situation I was in.

She didn't hesitate.

"You can come and cook whatever you buy at my place!" she said.

On Wednesdays, though Pierre didn't have a

holiday and could eat in the canteen as usual, there was no school for the younger two. I worked very early in the mornings, and in the evening after office hours; but I had some time free during the day. So I said to Pierre:

"On Wednesdays you can leave your brothers asleep when you go to school. I'll come back and see to them when I've finished my morning's work."

So that's what I did. I did my shopping on the way home and then gave the boys their cold-water breakfast. And then, as they couldn't stay shut up in the room all day, I took them with me when I went round to Emilie's to do the cooking. We'd eat part of what I made for our lunch, I'd keep a little bit for my own dinner, and the rest of it was set aside for the three boys' evening meal. At about four in the afternoon I'd leave Emilie's place to go back to work. I couldn't get away again to take the little ones back to the hotel, but I didn't have to worry: Pierre would come and collect them from Emilie's on his way back from school. Our system worked very well.

In the evening, when the children got hungry, they could eat what I'd set aside for them that morning. By then I was hungry too. I didn't want to spend money in the canteen, so I used to find a quiet corner and eat my share of the family meal there.

Saturdays and Sundays were difficult. Emilie often went away for the weekend, and when she did I couldn't follow the Wednesday routine.

"You can come and do your cooking early on Saturday morning," she'd say if she was going away.

"We won't be there for the rest of the weekend."

It so happened that on Saturday I only worked in the evening. So I used to hurry round and do my cooking in the morning, and go back to the hotel carrying our meals for the weekend. The children would have been waiting for me in our room. But after breakfast we had to go out, we weren't supposed to stay there during the day. That was the worst thing of all.

I often used just to draw the curtains and switch off the light to make people think we were out. We didn't leave our key at the desk. I'd have a word beforehand with the friendly chambermaid.

"I don't know what to do with the children over the weekend. The lady I leave them with on Wednesdays isn't there, and we can't walk around all day. If the boss asks about us, would you just tell him we're out?"

"Don't you worry," she said. "He won't know a thing."

So the children and I used to hide in the room for hours, without moving or making a sound, without even turning on the television.

We even had to eat our meals cold. When I got back to the hotel after doing the cooking at Emilie's I used to put the food in the refrigerator to keep it from going off. It had to last till Sunday evening. I did try to warm it up later by putting it in a saucepan and running the tap over the outside. But the water was never hot enough to make much difference.

The children hated it. Our sort of cooking uses

lots of oil and tomato sauce, and when it's cold it goes all sticky. But what could I do?

I tried to tell the boys it was better to eat even that than go hungry, but Tshakua only said:

"But, Mum – it's horrible!"

"I know," I said. "But if you don't eat anything today you'll be too weak to do any work at school tomorrow."

Sometimes he'd sulk.

"I'd rather have just a crust of bread. I'll have something to eat tomorrow in the canteen."

"No," I protested. "You must have a hot meal."

"But it's not hot – it's cold!"

He was right, but I wasn't going to give in.

"Yes, but it's got vitamins in it. It's better for you than just bread."

I'd go on scolding, and in the end he did as he was told. But even when we put each piece of meat under the tap to wash the grease off, it still tasted awful. But I knew the children, especially Tshakua, needed as much nourishment as they could get.

Thank heaven for the school canteen during the week! As for me, as often as not I just had a sandwich for lunch. Then someone told me there were places where I could get a meal for five or ten francs. I made inquiries, and found out there was one of those popular restaurants near the Porte de Clichy, patronised chiefly by Senegalese. So I went there and handed over my money – and I didn't like the food at all! It tasted quite different from our sort of cooking. But I had no choice. So not only did

I eat the meal I was given – I also asked them to wrap another one up for me for the evening.

I even brought some of it home for the children, but they wouldn't touch it. The Senegalese put something in their food that makes it smell, though not taste, very pungent. And our staple vegetable at home is rice, whereas I don't even know the name of what they eat most of in Senegal.

The children don't even like Rwandan cooking much. They will eat it when I give it to them, but not any more of it than they have to. They prefer what they get in the canteen, because they're used to it; they've always eaten French food. But that Senegalese stuff was different again, and they refused to touch it.

I had no choice, myself. I couldn't afford to cook for myself every day as well as for the children. I had to pay for the hotel and try to provide a few extras like bread, butter and something for the boys' tea. I didn't earn enough to go round.

Every Sunday I'd prepare the breakfast, and then at about ten o'clock we'd get ready for church. Going to church is a great joy. You see the people you know, you hear the good word, and often words of consolation too. I used to forget some of my troubles there. Sometimes I'd even find myself laughing, I was so happy to see my fellow-countrymen again. And some of the things the minister said used to restore my courage.

I belong to a Protestant religion called the Pentecostalists. I love the services. First you kneel down and pray, say how sorry you are for your sins and weep. Then anyone who wants to bear witness gets up and speaks. For example:

"I wish to bear witness to God's goodness: I had such and such a problem, and He came to the rescue and solved the problem in such and such a way..."

It's very moving. Everybody thanks the Lord for all His blessings and lifts up his arms to glorify God. Then we dance and hop about and sing His praises. And after the witnessing the minister reads us a chapter from the Bible and preaches a sermon on it. Then they pass the plate round for the collection, and it's all over.

It always did me a lot of good, but I didn't know where to take the children afterwards. I couldn't go back to the hotel because the owner lived there. He'd seen us go out, and would be on the watch for us to go back. I had to find somewhere, some shelter, where we could spend the day. But where? With whom?

If I asked someone, "Brother or sister, are you going home now?" they always answered, "No, Sorry!"

They were all afraid that if they asked me home I'd stay on for ages or ask them to do something for me. So they all turned away. During the service, in church, we were glad to be together. But as soon as church was over it was every man for himself again.

"I'm not going straight home – I've got an appointment!"

"Afraid not – I have to go to the hairdresser's!"

They all wanted to be rid of me now. Three

children is too much of a good thing. There was nothing they could do for me.

So I used to hang around for a while near the church, and then we'd go for a little walk. The children had friends in the neighbourhood because we'd lived there when Pierre was small. Lots of members of our community live there still.

"Mum," one of the boys would say. "I'd like to see if I can find So-and-so."

"All right! Let's try!"

So we'd walk around the streets a bit, and sometimes they'd meet other children and lark about together, and a little time would go by. But then their friends would have to go home, and I'd take my children to the railway station. We'd sit on a bench on the platform and watch the trains go by and the people coming and going. Sometimes the children would run about and play, but after a while they'd come back to the bench and we'd all sit there together, bored stiff. Sometimes it was very cold and I'd get fed up and take the children on the train with me to Paris. I had a season ticket and it made the time go faster. Then, when it was almost time for dinner, we'd go back to Saint-Denis and the hotel.

Never in all my experience have I suffered as much as I did then. Never have I led such an awful life.

I wanted to see the social worker to explain the situation and made an appointment for her to come and see me. She asked how much I was paying and wanted to see the receipts.

"The problem is," she said, "you're living in a hotel. If you were in a flat you could apply for housing benefit. But the bills say 'hotel rental for four people,' so it wouldn't be any use my asking. The only solution would be for me to have the children taken into care."

Of course I wasn't having that. I reminded her that the reason why I was living in the hotel at all was so as to keep the children with me.

She said I was being obstinate, and left me a phone number on a piece of paper. When I got tired of being stubborn I could ring that number at any hour of the day or night and someone would come and collect the children.

"All right," I said, "I'll manage on my own. As long as I've got work I can cope. All I ask you to do is find me somewhere to live! Somewhere where I can feed the children properly and don't have to drag them about from pillar to post as I'm forced to do now."

She didn't hold out much hope.

So we went on living in the hotel. I always paid the rent on time as soon as I got my wages. I made my calculations: so much for the hotel and then, out of the five hundred francs left over, so much for my season ticket and the rest for incidentals. When the money was all gone, I just gritted my teeth and hung on. So long as the children were getting enough to eat I was prepared to stick it out till things got better. But it was difficult. Sometimes I had to run up a bill or two. I tried to see it through by just carrying on as we were, by keeping to the same routine, with all its problems, including what to do with the children at the weekend. As for myself, I didn't care.

And then one day...

We were really only supposed to sleep in the hotel, but with four mouths to feed I used to keep some provisions hidden away. I had to.

One morning when the chambermaid, the woman who'd been such a help to me before, was cleaning the room, she found a cockroach. Where had it come from? It's true there were a few breadcrumbs and such like lying about. Anyway, there it was: a cockroach came crawling out of the cupboard. And the chambermaid went and told the proprietor.

"Look what I've found!" she said.

He was furious.

It was late and quite dark when I got home that evening, but he was watching out for me and called me back as I was going up the stairs.

"I was willing to help you out for a while," he said, " but now it's all over. You've got to leave. Something has happened that I can't overlook."

"What's the matter?" I asked. "Have the children been naughty?"

"It's nothing to do with the children. It's you! We agreed from the start that you wouldn't stay in the hotel during the day and you wouldn't eat or do any cooking in your room. And now what do I find? Bread, meat, and heaven knows what besides. You've been bringing food in and keeping it there. And to top it all, a cockroach! If you'd left the room as you found it this would never have happened. Do you expect me to risk losing my other guests? Today there's just one cockroach in just one room – but the beastly things have got legs, haven't they? I was taking a risk, letting you have the children here at all. And now this! I don't say you don't pay regularly. You do. But I can't have you here any longer."

I tried to argue.

"But where am I to go?"

He wouldn't listen.

"You must just manage as you did before. You came here without any warning, and you can leave the same way. Don't ask me where you can go to – it's nothing to do with me!"

"Please! Try to see my point of view! I had to do something to feed the children!"

"I know. And if this had been the kind of hotel where they let rooms out by the month it would have been different. But I don't want trouble with the inspectors because of the children, and I don't want to lose my other guests because of the cockroaches! I want you out of here by tomorrow!"

It was the last thing I wanted to hear. I went up to our room.

I'd let Pierre sleep in the bed while we were in the hotel. I slept on the floor. Tshakua and Sango both wet the bed sometimes and I didn't want any trouble, so I used to spread a sheet of plastic on the floor with a blanket over it, and I slept there with the two younger ones on either side of me.

That evening Pierre realised something was wrong as soon as I opened the door.

"What's the matter, Mum?"
"We have to leave here tomorrow."
"But where can we go?"
"That's the problem!"

I explained why the owner of the hotel was throwing us out. We couldn't go back to Sylvie's place, either.

"So what are we going to do, Mum?"

I hadn't any idea. I thought for a bit.

"Tomorrow we'll just carry on as usual. I'll go to work, and you three boys are to go to school. When I come home I'll see how everyone's taking it."

So that's what we did. I set off for work as usual, Pierre left for college and Tshakua went to school, and Sango waited in the room for the chambermaid to come and drive him to the kindergarten before starting her day's work.

When I'd finished work in Paris I hardly dared come home. I knew I had to, but I was afraid. In the end I took the train out to Saint-Denis at about two in the afternoon. The owner of the hotel was in his usual place.

I said good-day. He said good-day. But he wasn't pleased.

I went upstairs. Opened the door. And there was Sango.

"Didn't you go to school?"
"No."
"Why not?"
"The lady didn't want to take me."
"And have you been here all day? Without anything to eat?"

He wasn't even five years old, and the only thing he'd had all day was water from the tap! I started to cry, and went down to see the chambermaid.

"You said you'd help me! And you left him there all day by himself!"

She was upset too.

"I would have taken him to school as usual, but the boss wouldn't let me. I have to do what I'm told here. He wants you to leave today. I haven't even done the room. He's going to have it disinfected after you've left."

But how could I take the children away without anywhere to go? I went to see the owner of the hotel to ask for more time. He wouldn't listen.

"My mind is made up. You've got to leave today. I've got the public hygiene people coming in tomorrow."

I started clearing up and putting our things in plastic bags. We hadn't got any suitcases. I was waiting for Pierre to bring Tshakua home from school. They came in at last, at about five. I ought to have gone to my evening work, but I couldn't leave without resolving the problem of what to do with the children.

"Pierre," I said, "I want you to take the younger ones and go round to Auntie Emilie's for the evening. I've got to go to work, but I'll come there too when I've finished. And don't worry – we'll sleep somewhere, even if we have to sleep in the street."

I phoned Emilie.

"Emilie, the children are coming round to your place to wait for me, and this evening..."

I didn't go into detail. I knew that if I did she'd say no, it was impossible.

"...this evening when I've finished work I'll come and fetch them."

"No problem," she said. "Only they'll have to come straight away because I'm just going out to work too."

So off we all went. As soon as Emilie saw the children with all the plastic bags she knew something was wrong.

"What's the matter?" she asked them.

Pierre told her the truth.

"Mum's gone to find us somewhere to live because we can't stay in the hotel any more. She told us to wait here. She'll come and fetch us this evening."

But Emilie's very quick on the uptake. She put down her key and said:

"I'll wait for your mother myself! You can see how small this place is. I've only got one room and I have to share that with my daughter. I've got a child too, you know!"

Pierre tried to reassure her.

"Don't worry! Mum'll be here!"

Meanwhile I, having started out late, got to work late, and was trying to get through my work as fast as I could. I was completely demoralised but I had to work – otherwise I'd never be able to make things any better. As I cleaned I tried to work out what time Emilie would get home. I didn't want to go there myself: it would only complicate things if she saw me. It would be best if I stayed in Paris and asked her over the phone to keep the children overnight: I'd have found a way out by the morning. I reckoned she ought to be home by nine o'clock. But when I rang up it was her husband who answered.

"Hello? I'd like to speak to Emilie."

She took over at the other end.

"Where are you calling from?"

"I'm still in Paris, at the place where I work. Emilie, I'm calling to ask you to keep the children for me tonight."

"Oh no!"

She started to yell.

I could hear her husband asking, "What are you shouting for?"

I could hear her answering him.

"They were at Sylvie's till she turned them out. Then they went to a hotel, and because I felt sorry for them I let her come here to do her cooking. And now..."

She'd got so angry that she'd hung up. I dialled again, and got her husband again.

"Please may I speak to Emilie?"

Emilie came on.

"Here I am, but you'll find the children outside. I haven't got room for them. Everyone's told you – the minister, everyone: you ought to hand the children over to the social services! But no – you won't give in! Too bad – you'll find the kids outside. I haven't got room for them."

"Let me talk to Pierre."
I tried to reassure him.

"I'm going to ring Adrienne and explain it's just for tonight. Then I'll call Emilie back. But you're not to move from where you are until I've sorted something out with Auntie Adrienne."

I'd thought of Adrienne because we prayed at the same church. But I knew she hadn't got a place of her own: she lived with her cousin.

"Listen, Adrienne," I said. "I want to ask you a favour just for tonight. I'm in Paris, and it's too late for me to get back to Saint-Denis. Will you have the children just for tonight? Please!"

"I'll have to ask my cousin first," she said, "and he's not back yet. You can phone back and ask him yourself in a little while, if you like."

"How long will he be?"

"Oh, he should be home in a quarter of an hour or so."

I rang Emilie's number again.

"May I have a word with Pierre, please?"

Pierre came on.

"I've talked to Adrienne," I told him, " but the man whose place she lives in isn't home yet. Try to keep Emilie quiet for a quarter of an hour or so, and when I've spoken to Adrienne's cousin you can all go round there."

I was still in the offices where I worked as a cleaner. There was no one else there. I switched the light off and waited. After twenty minutes I dialled Adrienne's number again. Engaged. I dialled again. Still engaged. At first I thought she must be making a call herself, but then I thought she must have left the phone off the hook. I couldn't think why. I kept calling back, but it was always engaged. In the end I realised what must have happened. I'd told Adrienne that the children were waiting at Emilie's, she'd rung Emilie, and Emilie had explained the situation. So, to avoid getting involved, Adrienne had deliberately left the phone off the hook.

I had to do something, or else Emilie would do as she'd threatened and turn the children out. I didn't know what to do. I plucked up my courage and spoke to Pierre again. The children knew where Adrienne lived and could find their way there without me. So they must go there. I'd spoken to her and she knew what was happening. Of course, I'd rather have had her cousin's permission first, but as I couldn't get through on the phone I had no choice but to force her hand. So:

"Pierre," I said, "I want you to take your brothers round to Auntie Adrienne's. I've spoken to her about it, Her cousin's still not back, but she'll tell him when he gets in. I'll come too to make sure everything is all right. Don't worry if he doesn't open the door straight away. Just wait. Have you got all that?"

I tried to call Adrienne again but the line was still engaged. So I set off back to Paris. First one train, then another. All the time I was imagining the children out on the landing. I didn't know where I was going to take them if Adrienne's cousin wouldn't put them up for the night. The journey seemed to take for ever. It felt as if Saint-Denis were on the other side of the world.

When I rang at Adrienne's door she let me in, and I found the three boys lying scattered around her sitting room. She had her own children to think of.

"I kept trying to get through to you on the phone, Adrienne," I said, "but –"

"Oh! Perhaps someone didn't put the receiver back properly! Anyhow, I spoke to my cousin but he wouldn't agree. We all have our problems of our own, Thérèse, and he's already putting me and my children up. And now you turn up with yours!"

I tried to plead my cause.

"Adrienne, it's only for tonight! I know I'll be able to sort something out tomorrow."

She started to shout.

"That's what you say! Everyone keeps telling you you ought to have the children taken into care, but no, you won't! And then the rest of us have to bear the brunt! What do you expect me to do?"

I tried to calm her down.

"Don't worry, it's only for one night. And thanks for finding somewhere for them to curl up! I was so relieved to find them asleep when I got here. And now I'd like to speak to your cousin."

"No, I'm not going to disturb him now. It'll have to wait till tomorrow. You can talk to him when he wakes up."

I turned to Pierre.

"You'll have to give your brothers their breakfast as best you can tomorrow. Here's a bag with the rest of the bread from this morning, the powdered milk and so on. No one's to go to school. I'll come straight here after I've finished my morning's work. Got that?"

"Right."

I left. Adrienne didn't even ask me where I was going to sleep.

It was after eleven. Almost midnight. The last bus had gone, and I had to rush to the station at Saint-Denis to catch the last train to Paris. I worked in the Air France offices in the evening, and one of the bosses there was a nice young man who stayed on till one in the morning. I'd arranged things with him earlier that evening.

"I'm going to have to spend the night here," I'd told him. "First I have to go to Saint-Denis to sort out something for the children. But I'll be back here before you leave."

Then I explained my plan.

"This is the only way I can manage. You can lock me up for the night in one of the offices where I do the cleaning. There isn't any money around to steal! I can sleep on a couple of chairs, and either you or one of your mates can let me out in the morning. The Air France shuttle buses start from here at five in the morning, so I can catch one of them to get to my morning job on time."

So that's what we did. He locked me in one of the offices till five the next morning.

Just before five I heard the key in the lock.

"Are you all right?"

It was one of the other Air France employees. The one who'd helped me last night had put him in the picture. I told him about why I'd had to sleep there, but he was nice and said it didn't matter. I went up to the ladies' room and washed. Then I went to work, and after that straight back to Adrienne's.

The children hadn't had anything to eat.

"Auntie Adrienne wouldn't let us," Pierre explained. "She has to do as her cousin tells her. He said, 'I don't mind you helping them out for one night but I'm not having them staying here. Don't let them do anything!' So I couldn't get the breakfast."

I pleaded with Adrienne.

"Just for – "

"No! No! You know this isn't my own place! I have to do as my cousin says. I've been waiting for you to come and take your children away. Now take them and go to – I don't know... anyone. There are plenty of us Rwandans in Paris. Some of them have got places of their own. Take your kids to one of them!"

"All right."

I told Tshakua to get ready to go. He hadn't been washed, and apart from his medicine, which Pierre had managed to give him somehow, he hadn't had anything to eat or drink. I couldn't help starting to cry, seeing them all in that state. But still...

"Come on, everyone!" I said. "Up you get!"

They all stood there holding our plastic

bags and waiting for me to decide what to do. I looked from one to the other. But especially at Tshakua.

"God!" I thought. "What are we paying for in this life? Why all this, why?"

I went and stood in the middle of the room.

"What's it all for?" I cried aloud. "God, if you exist – what is it for? Where am I to go? I can't see a way out any more. These poor children will have to be taken into care. And then what will become of Tshakua? Where can we go?"

I stood there motionless for about ten minutes, trying to think. Going over everything in my mind.

When the bailiffs came and threw me out we went and spent one night at the minister's. He asked Sylvie to take us in. Then Sylvie threw us out. And now this business of the cockroach in the hotel...

All our troubles began because of Kasongo. I've thought and thought about it, but I've never been able to understand why he did that to me. We might at least have discussed what to do about Tshakua! But he left without saying anything. He left me without a penny, without any means of coping, without a job or anywhere to live. I had nothing, he was the one who went out to work, and he left without warning, without even leaving his address. I'm sure he thought that when I was left on my own I'd have to let Tshakua be taken into care. And it's true that if God hadn't given me so much strength Tshakua would probably be living with some other family by now.

But I'd made up my mind. Even if I didn't know where I was going to sleep that night, even if Tshakua and I were going to have to sleep in the street, I intended to fight, and I have fought.

Still, that morning at Adrienne's I felt as if I'd reached the end of my strength. I'd tried to get help from a friend, I'd tried staying in a hotel. Everything had failed. What door was there left to knock on? Then suddenly I had an inspiration.

"Come on, children," I said. "We're going to the town hall. It's our only hope,"

"There we'll go and there we'll stay. It doesn't matter if they throw us out of the office – we'll camp outside in the courtyard. And we won't go away till they find us somewhere to live."

Pierre didn't like this idea.

"But, Mum, you'll make yourself look ridiculous! People don't do that sort of thing!"

But my plan was growing clearer in my mind, and I knew I was on the right track.

"Maybe I shall make myself look ridiculous! But we're going to squat in the town hall, plastic bags and all!"

And that's exactly what we did.

I knew the town hall very well. I'd gone there after Kasongo left me, to apply for somewhere to live. But they sent me away.

"You need at least three wage slips. For three consecutive months. Otherwise I can't do anything for you."

I didn't wait three months. I applied straight away to all the likely organizations I could think of:

AIDES, APPART, SOLIDARITE-ENFANTS-SIDA.[†]

None of them could do anything for me. I even wrote to the President of France, but he never replied. I was reduced to writing threatening letters. "...If you don't find something for me I'll kill myself and take my children with me. It's a disgrace! I'm forced to live in a hotel where I'm not allowed to cook for the children even in the middle of winter! If you don't find me somewhere to live where I can cook properly I shall come to your office and kill first my children and then myself."

Of course I didn't really mean it. I'm a Christian – I'd never do such a thing in any circumstances. But I had to threaten them to make them listen. And I was distraught I couldn't get anyone to do anything. My only consolation was to tell my troubles to someone. The only way I could get anyone to do anything was to shout and cause a scene.

I gradually realised that as I couldn't get anywhere with his officials my only real hope was the mayor himself. So every now and again I'd go to the town hall and ask to see him. I was always told I couldn't see him without an appointment. But time went by and they never gave me an appointment. And now here we were!

"It's gone on long enough!" I thought. "Either

[†] These are three of the many French national organizations dealing with AIDS. AIDES is a large group with branches all over France, working to prevent AIDS and help its victims. APPART concentrates on housing and social rehabilitation. SOLIDARITE-ENFANTS-SIDA aims particularly at helping children affected by AIDS.

they find us somewhere to live this very day, or tonight we sleep in the town hall!"

So I took my Tshakua and the others, and off we went. And instead of stopping in the administrative offices downstairs I went straight up to the mayor's own office on the first floor. There I sat myself and the three boys down on the floor outside the mayor's door, with Tshakua's bottle of medicine in my handbag and all our luggage around us.

Up came a receptionist to shoo us away.

"You're not allowed to come up here!"

"Maybe not, but I'm going to stay!. I want somewhere to live! I know there are lots of empty houses. And I realize you can't just give them away. But I'm all alone with three children to look after, and I'm at the end of my tether!"

"You must go and see your social worker."

"I've been to see her hundreds of times and nothing has come of it. Now the town hall's got to solve the problem – I want you to find me a place where I can cook for my children."

She asked me to explain. I told her the whole story.

"... I've got the three monthly pay slips they ask for. I've had them for ages. But I've never had any reply to my applications for housing – I don't even know the reference number of my file! I kept on going in to inquire, but no one took any notice of me. I've written several times to the mayor telling him how I spent all I earned on the hotel and couldn't always afford to feed the children. And asking him to see me. But I suppose he put all my letters at the bottom of the pile."

I could see she was beginning to understand. I pressed on.

"But now he's got to take notice! I'm out on the street! All I ask is for you to phone the man who owns the hotel and ask him to keep me on till I can find somewhere more suitable. And meanwhile to arrange for me to do some cooking and keep some food in reserve, just like anybody else. Or else you must find somewhere else for us to sleep tonight. Here's the phone number of the hotel. All you have to do is arrange things with the owner. I'm quite prepared to pay... And if you don't do something I'm staying here!"

"You can't do that! Think of the scandal!"

"Well, where do you want me to go?"

"Haven't you got any friends?"

"I've tried that. They're fed up with us. It's been going on too long."

She started talking about the social worker again.

"I've told you already – there's no point! The only thing she can suggest is taking the children into care."

"Well, that's the best solution!"

She was getting on my nerves.

"No, it isn't the best solution! I don't want to be parted from my children! So either you arrange things with the hotel or I stay here."

"But you can't do that! You're in the way!"

"I'm not in anyone's way. Not so much as if I

was out on the street like a beggar instead of in here in the warm! And this evening, when you shut the place up and go home, I'll go out in the courtyard till the morning. I'm living here from now on! Everyone will be able to sleep sound, including me. And I shan't be in anyone's way."

And there I stayed, with the receptionist, outside the mayor's office. There were plenty of chairs around, but I preferred to sit on the floor. I set out all my bags and baskets around me. It made a fine spread. Sango and Tshakua sat there with me, but Pierre was embarrassed and went a little way off. He thought we were making fools of ourselves.

Time went by. Nothing happened.

After a while I asked the children if they were hungry.

"Yes!"

I gave Pierre some money.

"There's a MacDonald's round the corner. Go and get yourself and your brothers some cokes and hamburgers and chips. And some bread."

When he came back they spread all the things out on the floor, and I broke the baguette and handed it round. There were crumbs everywhere! You should have seen the mess! The receptionist was horrified.

"You're turning the place into a pig-sty!"

"What can I do?" I said calmly. "They were hungry. They didn't even have any breakfast today. Children have to eat, you know."

"But they make such a noise!"

"I can't help that!"

"You might at least tell them to keep quiet!"
"All right!"
I called the boys over.
"Make a noise!" I whispered.
I knew what I was doing, but Pierre was worried,
"She'll say the kids are being a nuisance!" he said.
"Don't worry about that!" I told them. "You just enjoy yourselves! Shout as loud as you like!"
You ought to have seen them! They just went mad! At last they could have some fun! It was because of the noise that Sylvie wanted to get rid of them. In the hotel it was even worse. And now I was actually ordering them to kick up a row! They didn't need telling twice!
The receptionist was furious.
"For heaven's sake! This is supposed to be an office! And look at all the litter – crumbs, chips, cans all over the place! That does it! You must go downstairs!"
"Certainly not!" I said. "And who are you to give me orders? I don't know you. But I do know you haven't any authority. If you had I expect you'd do something for me! But it's the mayor who has the power. And he knows all about me – I've written to him often enough. I've even come up here a few times to try to see him. And every time you made me fill in a form about who I was and what I wanted. But I don't know what you did with them. Threw them away, I suppose."
"I did no such thing!"
"That means you don't count – you have no

power! But the mayor's got power, and he knows why I'm here! And if when he comes out of his office he just tells me to go away, I'll go down and sit in the courtyard until someone solves my problems."

"Look, suppose some members of Parliament had an appointment this afternoon? What would they think? All those chips and bits of I don't know what! Come on now – go downstairs and sort things out with the social services people."

"No. There's no one down there with the power to make decisions. Only the mayor can do that. And I won't go downstairs until he's made some."

And there I sat. She wasn't at all pleased, and went to fetch the mayor's secretary.

"What's going on?" said the secretary. "We can't have this! Call the police!"

She was trying to scare me. She didn't know me.

"Yes, you call the police!" I said. "I'm waiting here until I get what I want. If you want me to leave, arrange for the hotel to have me back. Here's the number. If we're talking about scandals, my children couldn't go to school this morning. And they didn't have any breakfast, either. That's something that ought not to be allowed. I work, I pay for my room, and now the owner of the hotel throws me out. What am I supposed to do?"

"You must go and see the social worker."

The old tune.

"You go and see her! She knows all about it. So

does the mayor. So does everybody. All I want is to have my problems solved."

I made another effort to make myself clear.

"You can push and shove. You can call the police. You can do whatever you like to try to get rid of me. But I've made up my mind not to budge."

At this point a lady I didn't know came upstairs with my file.

"Would you kindly come down to my office?" she said.

"No, madam, I won't come down to your office. I'm not in anyone's way here."

"Yes you are!"

"No! You're in our way – in my children's way! This building belongs to the state, and I live in this country: I have rights the same as anyone else. If anyone killed me the state would have to put him on trial. It's the state's duty to protect me. And yet we can't eat properly, we haven't got anywhere to live, and the children haven't had their breakfast. So to all intents and purposes you're killing us. Why are you allowed to get away with it? When somebody commits a murder the state is supposed to try him. Well, here I am in a state building, and here I stay until I get satisfaction."

But this lady was different from the others.

"I'm sorry," she said. "I can't have made myself clear. I've been sent up here especially on your account. Look, this is your housing file. The mayor has been informed: it was his secretary who asked me to come up. I'm the person in charge of your file. You didn't meet me when you made your application, but I'm in charge of all the housing files. And the mayor has asked me to see him about your case. So please go down and wait for me. My name's on this card – please go and wait in my office while we study your problem."

"All right," I said. "You have my file and I believe what you say. But I warn you – if you don't come up with a solution you'll see me back here again!"

So down I went and someone showed me the way to her office. I left the children there and went to a phone just opposite. I had the telephone numbers of the lady who worked for AIDES and of some anti-racist organisation where they'd told me they'd written to the mayor and were following up my case. I also had the number of TF1, the television channel. Their offices were in the same building as those of Air France, and I knew some women who worked there. They'd told some of the TF1 people about me and I'd been give a number to ring if the occasion arose.

I called up all these numbers.

"I'm at the town hall, " I told everybody. "The person responsible for my file is with the mayor now, discussing my case. Please phone up and remind them of all the details – the fact that I've got children, that we haven't got a roof over our heads, and so on."

"I'm at the town hall," I told TF1. "If my problem hasn't been solved by the time office hours are over, could you come and film me here?"

They said they would, and gave me a number

where there was someone on duty around the clock.

I called the lady at AIDES, who'd also written to the mayor on my behalf, and asked her to support me. She promised to phone straight away.

Then I went back to the lady's office and waited. She'd told us to stay there, so I did, and after a good half-hour had gone by she came back.

"You really are something!" she said. "Your problem's solved. People have been ringing up from all over the place about you, and the mayor decided to take a personal interest in your case. So we don't even want to know how much you earn; we're not even investigating your situation; we're just making decisions and seeing they're carried out at once. And the result is you're being sent to a hotel. We'll phone there right away, and you're to go and stay there until we've found you a flat."

They were going to send me to a hotel in Paris, free of charge! It was in the boulevard de Rochechouart. There was one room for the children and another one for me – and we wouldn't have to pay a single franc! I was very pleased, of course, but worried too.

"Yes, that's all very fine, but what about the children? I have to work. How are they going to get from a hotel in Paris to their schools in Saint-Denis right out in the suburbs?"

They reassured me.

"That only goes to show this is just a temporary arrangement. Children aren't allowed to miss school for long. In a few days from now, a week or two at most, your situation will be sorted out once and for all."

"Thank God!" I thought.

So the mayor's secretary phoned the hotel to say we were on our way. Then she told me about a place near the Anvers metro station which provided various services, including a restaurant, for Jewish children. From there, she said, I could get vouchers entitling the children to free meals. I could give them breakfast in the hotel if I wanted to. I could cook there as much as I liked. But as I was short of money she suggested we should go to this restaurant for our main meals.

Then she gave me the address of the hotel and said:

"We'll be in touch with you about the flat."

We stayed in the hotel for some time. Pierre went to his usual classes at Saint-Denis, but Tshakua and Sango stayed with me: their old schools were too far away. In the morning I took them with me to work. I had no one to leave them with, and I couldn't have worked all day worrying about them shut up in their room on their own. I woke them up early, got them ready, and off we went. After I'd finished work in the morning we went and had lunch, and then I took them back to the hotel. I spent the early part of the afternoon with them, then they both stayed quiet for a while until Pierre got home, and I went off to do my evening's work. And so the time went by.

Then one fine day I was summoned to the town hall.

"We've found you somewhere to live," they said.

It was here in Saint-Denis – the flat we're still living in now. I can't find words to express how delighted we were with it – Tshakua, Pierre and I. We didn't know what to say. The whole place had been done out, complete with new wallpaper and fitted carpets. Even the sink and the bath were new. I hadn't expected anything like this! The biggest surprise for me was how large it was. In my application for accommodation I'd only asked for the minimum – a three-roomed flat with one bedroom for me, another for the children, and a living-room. And they'd given me four rooms. With a big balcony, too, where you could sit outside in the summer. And it was so clean! I didn't have to do anything but just move in. It was the end of a long nightmare that had been going on since 1988, when Kasongo left me. It was 1990 by the time we had a home of our own again at last.

*

They were the worst two years of my life. Three weeks here, a fortnight there, then the hotel, and never any peace, never any possibility of being like an ordinary family and leading a normal life. And I'd had to learn to lie: all that time I was for ever trying to invent excuses, always having to hide, always afraid of being found out. Even with friends, people who were supposed to like me, I had to resort to all sorts of tricks when it came to giving Tshakua his medicine.

"Come along, dear, let's go out for a breath of fresh air, shall we?"

It was the only way open to us; there was no other solution. But for two whole years! That's a long time. And all because I'd made up my mind never to be parted from my child.

And he was ill, too. The school was always sending for me.

"What's the matter with him?" they'd ask.

"Nothing! Nothing whatsoever!"

If ever there was a germ around, Tshakua was bound to catch it. He's the sort of kid who catches everything! And whenever that happened I had to lie and pretend he was just a normal child. It was very difficult, because at that time he was always getting ill. Especially in the winter, when he played outside with the other children during break. I couldn't ask the teachers to give him special treatment. I wanted them to treat him just like the rest. But when the weather was cold or when it snowed it was too much for him: he got swollen glands and a temperature and was always in bed or even in hospital. So naturally he was often away from school.

Some people might think all I had to do was let the teacher into the secret. But she was just an ordinary woman and would have reacted the same way as everyone else. I wanted the other children to treat Tshakua like one of them, too. And so I had to lie, everywhere and all the time, at the school and among our friends, wherever Tshakua went.

I still have the same problem: as far as that's concerned, nothing has changed. And it's not easy, because I've been taught not to tell lies. It makes me feel guilty, and yet I'm forced to do it. But still, I think I'm right: they're good lies, and I'm doing my duty as a mother when I tell them. It's thanks to them that Tshakua has friends and fun and some pleasures in life. It's thanks to them people don't point the finger at him. It's our secret, his and mine and our family's. I tell lies in the same way as I once stole, the day when it was the only thing I could do. I had thought to myself, "I don't want the children taken away from me because they're not getting enough to eat. I don't want them taken into care for the lack of anything." And if I had to steal so that they could eat, too bad! Even if I'd been taken to court I could have explained how there was no canteen on Wednesdays. So I wasn't doing wrong. On the contrary. I felt better stealing than begging in the metro. Deep down inside I knew I wasn't a beggar. I did an honest day's work, I did all I could, with all my courage and all my strength, but I had to pay for the hotel, and that day there was nothing left to buy a bit of meat for the children.

Oh dear, it is difficult! The times I've wept about it all! And I even had to hide to do that, just as I had to hide to give Tshakua his medicine. Always hiding. But what else was I to do, in the circumstances, if I wanted my son to be happy?

One day Tshakua was round at a neighbour's

place: it's very bad for a child to be shut up all the time on his own, especially if he's got health problems already. Sango wasn't living with us any more by then: soon after I moved into the flat my brother found a job and a house, so he sent for his wife and they took their son back again. I was still on my own, and working. When Pierre wasn't studying he was starting to go out with his friends. So after school Tshakua used to go and wait for me at this neighbour's house. It was winter, and cold, and it got dark early. And then one day I got home from work and found him standing there on the landing!

"What's wrong?"

"It's Auntie Antoinette's husband – he says I'm not to go there any more!"

"Why? Have you been naughty, Tshakua?"

"No, Mum – I swear I haven't!"

"But you must have done something, darling, for them to turn you out! For a grown-up person with a family of his own to turn you out on a cold night like this! There must have been some reason!"

I almost went round straight away to ask for an explanation, but I was too upset. I decided to wait until I met them. And the first time I saw Antoinette I went up to her.

"Antoinette," I said, "I have to be at work a lot of the time, and now Pierre's older he goes out, he has girlfriends, he's not often at home. That's why I sent Tshakua round to play at your place. What did he do that made you turn him out like that?"

She started mumbling some complaint or

other, and wouldn't look me straight in the eye. Then she said:

"It wasn't me who told him he wasn't to come round any more. It was my husband."

"And what did you think about it?"

She was very embarrassed,

"You know, Thérèse, there's no arguing with my husband. I did remind him that Tshakua's only a little boy and you're all on your own... But he wouldn't listen. So I tried – "

"But in the end you threw him out? Even though it was dark?"

She didn't know what to say.

"It isn't me – it's my husband."

Afterwards, thinking it over, I realised Tshakua hadn't really misbehaved. So I asked him:

"Have you ever taken your medicine when you're round at Auntie Antoinette's?"

He was on AZT then.

"Sometimes. If I haven't taken it here before I go."

Then I understood. Children don't think to hide anything, and Antoinette's husband had probably come across the medicine bottle. And so, to protect his own children...

"But Tshakua, I told you you must always take your medicine before you went there!"

But it was too late.

CHAPTER THREE

My own choice

I haven't got a lot of photographs because I don't take many, and most of those I had I've taken back to Rwanda. But I have found one that dates from when I first started looking after Tshakua, when he was still in the crèche. It was taken in his room there. He was only eight and a half or nine months old – he hadn't started to walk yet. I used to go and see him at the weekends. There he'd be in his cot, stretching out his little arms to me. He had such wonderful big black eyes, and skin so fair. And whenever I left him I could hear him calling me as soon as I got out into the corridor: "Mummy, Mummy!" Poor little soul, shut up all alone in his room! In Africa a baby's always surrounded by grandmothers and aunts, nieces and cousins. There's always someone to pick him up or play with him, because out there we don't stay at home all the time – we keep moving about. When it's time for a baby to be fed, either its mother comes to it or someone takes it to her. But the rest of the time it's just as likely to be left with the other women. Here in Europe it's quite different: a mother has to look after her baby herself and be with it all the time. But back home all the family live within reach and just take it in turns.

So little Tshakua, who back in Rwanda had been used to having people coming and going around him all the time, was now stuck in a room by himself, like all the other babies in the crèche. So when he couldn't see me any more he'd start calling out "Mummy, Mummy, Mummy!" as if he was never going to stop. I didn't have the heart to go, then. I'd start to cry myself, and couldn't help going back to give him another cuddle.

He must have thought I was all the family he had, because apart from me the only people he saw were strangers. And white people, at that. During the first few months of his life he hadn't even seen a white person! And I noticed that if a nurse came to change him, or if I called one of them in for anything, he'd cry and call out for me even when they picked him up

I've got another photograph, of myself and Kasongo and some friends. Kasongo was my friend; we adopted Tshakua together. It's a snap taken while we were in Brussels for a few days. It was the first time I'd ever been away on holiday with Tshakua. It was like a real family holiday, the kind you dream about.

When Tshakua was still in the crèche I didn't think of anything but the difficulties: how to find time to go and see him, how to get him out of the crèche, how to organize our own life so that we could take care of him. But when we started buying the flat and they let us have him with us, then we started thinking about holidays. So we hired a car and went away for a week. We stayed with friends, people from back home. They thought Tshakua was a lovely little boy – very sweet and intelligent.

Here he loved everybody. He'd let anyone pick him up, even people he'd never seen before. He'd laugh and chatter with them as if he was quite at home. He was glad to be alive again. His health was still good then. He didn't have any symptoms and didn't have to take any medicine.

The medicine came later. The doctors were always doing tests, one after the other. Even when he was still in the crèche, one of the assistants used to take him to the hospital for regular check-ups because they knew he was HIV-positive. And one day they had to begin the treatment.

When I started talking about adopting him, the professor in charge of his case asked me to go and see him.

"It's a very important decision," he said. "You must think it over seriously before you commit yourself."

"I've thought it over already," I said. "He's my child and I'm going to take care of him."

"Yes, you want to adopt him now. But what about afterwards? If his condition ever worsened it would be too late then to change your mind."

"I've already thought about that. I know all I need to know. You've told me he's HIV-positive – he's got the same illness as his mother. I know all that. But I still want to have him."

Perhaps they thought I'd regret what I'd let myself in for when I found out how difficult it is to bring up a child who's HIV-positive. They did all they could to warn me. They sent for Kasongo and me several times, and every time they asked us if we were still of the same mind.

"It's a very serious illness. A patient's condition may get worse from one day to the next. And we don't know how to treat the disease yet."

We knew all that quite well, but it didn't matter to us.

"I'm very fond of this child," I told them. "I've loved him from the very first time I saw him. I didn't know then that his mother was very ill, or that what she had was AIDS, or that it could turn out the way you say it can and she might die. But my heart went out to him already, I loved him already, anyway. He's my child and I want to keep him."

In the end they agreed to let us have him. We did all that was asked of us – bought a flat, provided a family background. All I was thinking of was Tshakua's happiness.

He loved it when he was five or six and started to go to school. He was very fond of his friends. But it was then that the difficulties began. He's quite well now, and please God make it last, but in those days he was very ill. From the time he was five or six he was always getting swollen glands and a temperature, and often he had to go into hospital. Especially in winter: it was just one earache after another. And when he was in hospital he kept asking when he could go back to school. We used to try to reassure him.

"You'll soon be better, but you must let yourself be looked after properly. You can go back to school as soon as you're well again."

The doctors explained things to me and gave me lots of advice. I knew his blood cells were very weak, so he couldn't protect himself and might catch all sorts of illnesses. The slightest sign of a temperature made me anxious. I was scared if anyone coughed near him. I knew everything was dangerous as far as he was concerned, and he's always been one of those kids that catch everything. Whenever he wasn't well or had a temperature or the least little thing wrong with him, Kasongo and I would both go crazy with anxiety.

"What's the matter? What's wrong with him?" we'd ask.

We'd been told so often they didn't know when the real illness would declare itself! But the doctor always answered:

"There's no change. It's just a bug... Nothing to worry about. It'll pass."

When Kasongo and I were both at work and Tshakua was by himself at home, I always used to phone to make sure he took his medicine at the right time and then waited for half an hour before eating anything.

"Have you taken your medicine, darling?"
"Yes, Mum."
"I'll ring back in half an hour and then you can have your lunch."

"Yes, Mum."

But one day when I was giving the house a good turn-out what should I find behind the refrigerator but all Tshakua's tablets! I cried and cried.

"How could you, my darling?"

I could hardly believe it.

"But, Mum, they taste nasty!"

"'Nasty'! And there was I phoning you every day to ask if you'd taken your medicine, and there were you saying 'Yes, Mum!'..."

And all the time he wasn't taking it at all!

Even now I can't be certain about his future. The doctors still say the illness could declare itself at any time, and we have to be prepared for it. They say that every time I see them. And so whenever he's ill I feel terrible myself. I love him so much, and I've loved him so long! I want so much to see him grow up!

"What about the miracle cure?" I ask the doctors who're always telling me anything might happen. "When are they going to find it?"

But there isn't any miracle cure, and whenever Tshakua's the least bit unwell I nearly die of dread. It's been like that ever since he was little, and gone on right up till now. It's overshadowed my whole life.

Various men have been interested in me, and I've tried several times to start a new life. But I've had a lot of disappointments because I've never known whether to tell or not. Would the man accept Tshakua if he knew?

One thing I do know. If a man doesn't love Tshakua he can't become part of my life.

MY OWN CHOICE

The choice I made, my decision to have my son to live with me, produced some negative results: men just couldn't understand it. They wanted me but not the child. Three men I've known have left me because of that, though in each case I had thought it was going to be all right.

The first time I thought someone loved me and we were going to have a family together was with Kasongo, Tshakua's "father". I was shattered when he went away. I realized I'd been mistaken: our relationship hadn't been the real thing. We'd lived as if we were a family, but he didn't really love me.

Still, we'd overcome all sorts of obstacles for the sake of the baby when people were making things difficult because we hadn't got anywhere to live. And he'd come with me to fetch Tshakua from the crèche. He'd known from the start that Tshakua was ill, and what was wrong with him – he was with me at the hospital when the doctor told me. But we looked for a flat just the same. We even went so far as to borrow money to buy one, because that was the only way we could have Tshakua to live with us straight away. And we didn't even have the right to any housing benefit!

So I'd thought Kasongo loved me, and that he was as keen as I was to give Tshakua a normal life. And in truth that's how it was at first, and Tshakua got very attached to him. He looked on Kasongo as his father, because he was the one who did everything for him. I was working all day, but fortunately Kasongo was prepared to help. We'd even bought a car, not for ourselves but for Tshakua. He was often ill and needed to be taken to a hospital in Paris instead of the local one, and sometimes it happened at night when there weren't any trains. So Kasongo took his driving test and we both saved up.

I used to leave the house before six in the morning to get to work by seven, and Kasongo, who didn't start work till later, always washed and dressed Tshakua and gave him his breakfast. Then he'd get a snack ready for him to take for his tea, and drive him to the day nursery. In short, Tshakua had a father.

And Kasongo and I really were happy. We got on well, we were very fond of one another, and Tshakua loved him too. When I got home in the evening I'd find Tshakua asleep on Kasongo's lap while he sat quietly watching the television, waiting for me to come in. I thought our love was going to last and that we'd have a real family. I even thought we were going to have a child together.

In our country, people are supposed to bring lots of presents when they visit a house where there's a new baby. And I'd noticed that whenever one of our fellow-countrymen had a child, Kasongo would grumble:

"We're always buying presents for other people's babies. When are we going to buy some presents for ourselves?"

So I said:

"I know you're very fond of Tshakua, and as you haven't got any children of your own, why don't we try to have a baby together, God willing."

We did try; but it didn't work. We both went

and had examinations, and my doctor told me I couldn't have any more children. I'd had one of my ovaries removed and it would be too difficult. He suggested we try *in vitro* fertilization.

I told Kasongo what the doctor had said and we decided to give it a try. We were very happy. Tshakua was still small and I knew he couldn't understand, but whenever we went to see a baby or one was brought to see us he was always very interested in it. So I told him I might be going to give him a little sister.

Tshakua was pleased and Kasongo was all for it, so I went through with the fertilization. At first it seemed to have been successful, I was pregnant! We were wild with joy, all of us. But there were complications. There was something wrong with the foetus and it had to be taken away. If I'd had it, it might have been still-born or handicapped.

I could have tried again but I had to rest first. I didn't desperately want another baby, but I wanted to protect the love between Kasongo and me and strengthen our marriage, because I thought Kasongo loved Tshakua and me and that we might have to face unhappiness later on. But eventually we gave up trying.

And then, all of a sudden, Kasongo left. Without so much as a thought for Tshakua. I could have understood it if he'd just stopped loving me or got another woman – but he'd been a father to Tshakua! I've known other couples who've parted. But even when the husband just sits down at the table and announces, "I'm leaving," he always goes

BELOVED SON

on to say, "What do you think we ought to do about the child?"

Kasongo knew I hadn't got a job. He could have said, "All right – I'll look after Tshakua until things get sorted out."

But no, he'd just packed his bag, put it in the car and driven off. I'd been out looking for work, and when I got back I found Tshakua standing outside the door with his medicine – he always took that with him wherever he went. Everything in the flat had been dumped on the landing. The bailiffs had sealed up the door. We hadn't even got a roof over our heads! I burst into tears and kept saying, "What am I going to do? No job, no money, and now nowhere to live!"

At first Kasongo and I had both contributed to the payments on the flat, but after a while I was working too hard and my health was failing, so we decided I'd just work part-time. This was when I still wanted to have a baby. I also felt I hadn't been spending enough time looking after Tshakua.

So as Kasongo was the only one with a full-time job, he was supposed to be paying the instalments on the flat. But, unknown to me, he'd fallen behind on the payments. He'd met his new girlfriend, and wanted to live somewhere else with her, so he just stopped paying. I found out afterwards that there'd been letters, final demands, suggestions for making other arrangements and so on. But they were all addressed to him, and I never opened his letters and he didn't say anything. By the time I found out that the flat had been sold it was too late to do anything. Otherwise I might have gone to see the social services, raised some money, or worked out a new agreement.

I kept going over and over all my troubles in my mind. My sister was dead. Tshakua was HIV-positive. I couldn't have any more children. I was tired and depressed. And now the bailiffs had come and thrown out everything I possessed. I thought of all this and wondered what on earth I was going to do.

I'd chosen Tshakua. If I hadn't done that I think our love might have lasted. Later on, too, I might have been able to keep the other men longer. But for me my son came before everything else. I wanted to give him more than the bare necessities. I haven't been blessed with many children, so my experience is limited. But in my opinion it isn't bringing a child into the world that creates the strongest bonds. It's bringing him up, devoting yourself to him completely day after day, sacrificing everything else to his needs and his happiness.

And the fact that a child isn't normal, that he's sick, that he's deprived because he hasn't got a mother, makes the relationship stronger still. When Tshakua calls me "Mum" I almost melt away with delight.

After Tshakua's "father" I met another man. We started to live together in my new flat, and I thought to myself, "I won't tell him too soon. Perhaps later. I don't even know yet if he's going to stay!"

So I tried to keep the truth from him. But he was living in my house, and Tshakua was still a child and didn't always think about hiding things. So one day this man found the hospital papers lying about, and the packet of AZT. That evening he was waiting for me when I got home from work. I came in carefree, happy and smiling, then noticed he looked worried and uneasy. He wouldn't look me straight in the eye.

"You know," he said, "I think we both ought to go and have a what-do-you-call-it – a check-up."

"What sort of a check-up?"

He jumped up, his teeth clenched.

"I want us to have some tests."

He loved me, I loved him, everything was going well. Then suddenly, I didn't know what was happening to me, but I felt as if something had just broken.

"He must have found the AZT," I thought, "and gone and asked somebody what it is."

He stood there facing me, trying to justify himself.

"We ought to get a general check made on our health. It's something everybody needs to know."

I shrugged.

"My own doctor does all the tests I need, and I go to the clinic regularly for smears! I'm perfectly healthy at the moment. So I don't see the point of having a check-up."

"Yes, but it's not a bad idea from time to time. Let's go. Please!"

I could see it wasn't as simple as that. I wished he'd just come out with it and say, "I've got problems, I don't feel too well. Something isn't working as it ought to and I'm worried." Or, "I've got a feeling there's something wrong with me. I'd like to go and check."

"Well," I said, "you may be worried, but I feel fine and am perfectly well."

He insisted.

"All right. But I'd just like you to come too."

I knew they wouldn't find anything. I agreed just to avoid bother. So we went to the hospital. I wanted him to come to my clinic but he wouldn't.

"No, no, we must go to such and such a hospital. They've got a special department."

A special department, eh? I understood but I wanted to make him say why he needed to go there.

"What sort of special department?"

"A screening unit..."

He was stammering now.

"I'm not feeling too well, you know," he said. "Before I knew you I went with many other women. So I'd like us to go and be tested..."

"What for?"

"AIDS."

So he knew. And he'd already made inquiries and found out where to go. As he didn't mention Tshakua, I didn't mention him either. So we went to the hospital and they gave us numbers: everything has to be done anonymously.

We got the results a few days later. Both negative. But that wasn't enough for him. He wanted everyone in the house to be tested. I drove him into a corner.

"But why? Tell me why!"

"Because I want to understand! Tshakua's always taking medicine – he never stops! What exactly is the matter with him?"

But I was beginning to get angry.

"You should have asked that before! First I have to go and have the test, but that's not enough for you. Now the children have to go too. But I know all about the state of their health: they don't need any more examinations. All you had to do, instead of making all this fuss, was to ask me straight out: 'Why does Tshakua have to take medicine sometimes?' If you'd asked I'd have told you."

"Well, tell me then!"

I looked straight at him.

"Yes, my son is ill. He's HIV-positive. So now you know."

"Oh!... Why didn't you tell me before?"

"Because I wasn't sure of you. We'd only just met. You couldn't expect me to tell you my whole life history straight away. But now you know. And it's up to you to accept it or not. Speak up – this is your home. You've only got to tell me what you think."

He knew Tshakua was another woman's child, but he was uneasy all the same.

"I've heard people say... I gather that if you live with anyone who's HIV-positive there are certain precautions... Tooth-brushes and so on... And if they bleed, you're not supposed to..."

Explanations, and yet more explanations! I couldn't stand any more of it.

"Listen," I said. "I'm going to work now, and I

don't want to find you here when I come back. You can leave the key in the letter-box. It's all over between you and me. If you can't live with Tshakua, too bad. I'm no different from you, and I'm not afraid. I've lived with him for years without worrying. If you're frightened, go! Take good care of yourself! Goodbye. I don't want to find you here when I come back."

I meant what I said. And that's what happened. When I came home I found his key in the letter-box.

"Oh well," I thought. "It's not that serious"

I've accepted everything for my son's sake.

Some time passed and I met someone else. I went to spend a few days with my brother and his wife in Douai, and we saw something of a man they knew called Manga. He worked there as an electrician. He was a bit older than me; about forty. He was bald, too, and that made him look older. But I liked him. So I said to myself, "I'm not going to make the same mistake twice. This time I'm going to warn him from the outset."

I asked him if he had any children.

He said he had.

"So have I. But one of them is ill."

"What's the matter with him?"

"He's HIV-positive."

"Since when?"

"Since he was born."

"Is he your own son? How did he get it?"

I told him everything.

"No, he's not my own son. He's my sister's. But

I look on him as my own. I love him as if he were my own. He is my son. I've looked after him since he was eight months old."

"I see. It won't be any problem. I love you as you are, with the life you have lived."

"Let's see if that's possible," I thought. But I took precautions anyhow before I started going out with him.

"I don't want you throwing it back in my face later on," I said. "Before you come and live with me I want us both to go and take some tests. You might already be ill without knowing it, and I don't want you coming to me and saying my son infected you. I'd rather be prepared for the worst."

He agreed, and we went to the same unit as the other man had taken me to. Again we were both negative.

"Right," I said. "So there's no risk of infection. If there were I'd have been HIV-positive long ago. So now just remember – there's no risk involved either for you or your children!"

He agreed, completely.

So we started seeing one another. As he worked in Douai he could only come to my place at weekends, and we got on very well.

But after a while he came to live with me. The man he worked for couldn't employ him full time anymore, so he moved to Paris. But it wasn't long before he took a sudden dislike to Tshakua. He seemed to look on him as a rival, someone to be crushed. He criticized him at every opportunity. One day he accused him of being rude because he hadn't said good morning. Another day it would be something else.

And one fine morning he told me:

"We ought to send Tshakua away to school."

"What for?"

"He's lagging behind in class and he'd work better at boarding-school. And he doesn't know how to behave. You spoil him. He'd learn to be more grown-up away from you."

"Your reasoning's all wrong. Since Tshakua was eight months old it's me that's looked after him, it's me who's his mother, and the first thing this child needs is to have his mother near him. How could you expect me to send him away to school. I could never take such a decision."

It so happened that this man was arranging for his own children to come over from Rwanda about then. His daughter Marie was already living with us. Before he met me, when he spent most of his time out of Paris, he'd left her in the country with a foster-mother, but since he'd come to Paris to work he'd taken the opportunity to have her back, and was very glad to have her living with him at my place. And now he was trying to separate me from Tshakua! But I was very firm.

"It seems to me you've got something against my son. You started by claiming he was rude and didn't say good morning. Then it was other things. And now you want to send him away from me. Well, I wouldn't bank on it if I were you! I was living with Tshakua when you met me, and you can leave us as you found us. Nothing on earth would make me part with him – just get that into your head!"

After that things started to go downhill. His little girl was slightly younger than Tshakua – she was about five or six and he was seven. And now her father started taking precautions on her behalf and making a fuss about the slightest thing. Mustn't do this, mustn't do that...

Next he wanted Tshakua to clean the toilet with disinfectant every time he went to the lavatory. The same when he had a bath. And he was supposed to remember all sorts of other precautions. I lost my temper.

"I've had enough! Before you came here I was leading a perfectly normal life, and no one fretted about every single thing that Tshakua did. But ever since you've had your daughter here, all you can think about is protecting her, and you're making our lives unbearable! I can't stand it any longer. You dislike Tshakua – I've known that for a long time. I can tell by comparing you with Kasongo. When Tshakua was eight months old, Kasongo and I adopted him together. Kasongo loved Tshakua and was a father to him all the time he lived with me. But you're starting to get on my nerves – all this nagging about boarding school and precautions to protect your daughter. I've had enough. A man who dislikes my son has no business here. You can go whenever you like!"

He left. Leaving Marie with me. The woman who'd been her foster-mother was living in Douai now and couldn't have her back, so her father asked me if I'd look after her until he found someone else. Of course I said I would, and I took care of her as if she were my own. She was a dear little thing, but rather sad after her father went away. She'd always been very close to him. Now she kept thinking about her mother, too, back in Rwanda. She was always talking to me about her and asking when she'd see her again. I gave her her meals and watched over her health and her progress at school. Then one day during the holidays, when I was out at work, he came and took her back. He'd been gone two or three months. I just came home one evening as usual and he'd taken her away. Without a word of warning. I looked for her everywhere, but he'd collected all her clothes and other belongings. I expected him to phone the next day or some time in the days that followed, but he never did.

The teacher asked me why Marie wasn't going to school any more. What could I say?

Then I met Ngenda, my present husband.

We went to the same church, and one day he began courting me. But my experience with Manga had taught me a lesson, so at first I didn't respond.

"You're very nice and serious and I know you're God-fearing because we met in church," I told him. "I'm sure you're a good man and wouldn't do anyone any harm. But I don't think I could try to start a new life again."

"Why not?"

I told him the truth straight away.

"I've got a problem."

"What is it?"

"I've got a child who's ill."

"What sort of illness has he got?"

"He's just ill. I don't want to say any more."

Ngenda had often met Manga. Manga didn't go to church himself, but he came and picked me up afterwards. Ngenda knew I'd lived with him.

"That's why Manga left me. He wouldn't accept my son any more, and I couldn't tolerate that. So I suppose my life as a woman will have to come to an end. Everyone's afraid. And if ever I did find another friend, he'd be sure to find out one day about my son. Then there'd be more trouble, and in the end he'd leave me too. I don't think it's worth it."

But Ngenda wouldn't let me off so easily. He was already very fond of me and he wanted to hear more. I don't know why, but I trusted him. And I longed to be able to talk to someone. Ngenda knew Tshakua already because I often take him to church with me. He liked the boy. So I told him everything.

"Well, Tshakua's got this illness. His mother died of the same thing. It's... " I said the word. "And that's why I think there's no point in hoping too much."

But Ngenda wasn't daunted in the least.

"I accept you just the same. And I accept Tshakua and his illness. Just wait and see! I'm a religious man, I go to church every Sunday. Let God be my judge if I lie. I ask you, on this Bible, to trust me."

He convinced me.

Tshakua had often met him before. They used

to talk together after church, and Ngenda played with him sometimes. He started calling him "Uncle" straight away.

"You've seen already how nice Uncle is. And now he's coming to live with us. I expect you realize I love him, so there's no point in trying to hide it."

Tshakua had already seen quite a few uncles come and go, but none of them had really been good to him. Now I tried to share my hopes with him.

"This Uncle's going to be your father. You can call him Daddy if you like. But whether you do or not, from now on he will be your father."

Tshakua was very pleased.

So Ngenda came to live with us. He was kind to Tshakua and Tshakua liked him. There was a pleasant atmosphere in the house, and we started to think about having a future together. Like me, Ngenda was no longer in his first youth, and he'd got children too. We were responsible people: why shouldn't we get married instead of living in sin? Our church doesn't allow cohabitation. So we made up our minds and went first to the town hall and then to the church to find out what we had to do. And on December 28th we were married.

It was a great day for me, a day that changed my life completely. It had never been as serious as this with the other men I'd loved: we'd lived as man and wife, but never felt any need to get married. But this time it was a real wedding, and we were a real couple who were going to stay together for ever. It was wonderful – something I'd been waiting for for a long time. But this was the first time I'd ever felt sure enough of anybody to make such a commitment. And he was eager to share his future with me. He accepted Tshakua in spite of his illness, and it didn't occur to him to make me have tests to see if I'd got AIDS. I truly believed he was made for me and would never leave me. Only God will ever separate us.

So we started to live as a real family.

We were a family from the beginning, because of Tshakua, and Pierre was still living with us too. But Ngenda had three children back in Rwanda. It was I who suggested they should come and live with us.

"Tshakua's always on his own," I said, "because I don't like sending him where there are children any more. Why don't we send for yours?"

Ngenda thought it was a good idea. He took the necessary steps, and the children arrived. So now Tshakua has some brothers and sisters. I've never seen him so happy. He doesn't have to spend whole days shut up watching television any more, and whereas he used to be sad at not being able to go out, now he doesn't even want to. They all play together in their room, and I can hear him laughing and having fun like other children. In the past he never went away for the weekend or spent a day with friends or anything – I didn't like to let him go anywhere without me. And I couldn't take him out very often myself; I don't earn much money. And of course he could never go away on holiday because he has to show up at the hospital once a fortnight. But now he has a nice cheerful life.

The only break he ever had, before, was going to Douai every so often to stay with my brother. It was the only holiday Tshakua ever had. I've always told my brother and his wife my troubles, but they never made a fuss about precautions. Tshakua was happy with them, and would have liked to go there more often.

But he doesn't even think about that any more. We're a family ourselves – my husband and his children, Tshakua and me – and life is easier now. Parents' meetings are always held at times when I'm at work, so my husband always goes. He goes to the hospital too, if I can't manage it. And every day we take turns in looking after Tshakua: Ngenda sees to his treatment in the morning, and I take over in the evening when I get home. Tshakua dislikes taking DDI[†], you see, and you can't rely on a child to do something he doesn't want to. Especially as it's very complicated now: he's supposed to go without food for two hours, then sip his medicine very, very slowly, then wait for another half-hour before having anything to eat. But we've got it all organized, and I can go off to work with an easy mind. The months go peacefully by, and I really think I'm glad, at last, to be alive.

What Tshakua has always lacked is a father. That's the only question he's ever asked me. He used to ask it often.

"Where is my father? Why don't I ever see him?"

† DDI is the drug didanosine, an anti-viral drug similar to AZT.

I've never been able to meet that need, and I could see it used to make him unhappy. He's never had a father who was always there, someone he could really rely on. He called me Mummy as soon as he started to talk: so he had a mother. He and I both used to visit his real mother sometimes, when she was in hospital: I used to fetch him from the crèche so that she could see him. But he called her Auntie; I was already his Mummy. Yet he's never said, "Mum, are you really my mother? And where is Auntie, that I used to know when I was little?" The only thing he's ever asked is who was his father.

I tried to explain.

"Lots of children don't have a father. You're one of them. Sometimes a mother's going to have a child and the father's not there any more – he left as soon as they found out about the baby, or else he decides later that he doesn't want the responsibility. But don't you worry – I'm your mother, and I've been a father to you as well. You haven't been deserted!"

Sometimes I'd add:

"If you really want a father we'll pray very hard, and perhaps one day God will send you one who'll adopt you."

That's the sort of answer I've always given him. But I know it doesn't satisfy him and that he goes on trying to find out the truth. He harps on the subject often. I can always tell what's bothering him when he says:

"So and so's father came and they did this, that

and the other. I wish my father would come one day and do things with me."

He makes up things at school, too. Once his teacher noticed and said to me:

"We know Tshakua hasn't got a father, but sometimes he tries to make us think he has. He says things like, 'Oh, I can't do that – my father said I wasn't to.'"

Tshakua used to call my brother Daddy when he first came to France. But later on he understood and started calling him Uncle. With Ngenda it's the same: sometimes calls him Daddy and sometimes Uncle. At first, though, before Ngenda's own children came, he used to call him Daddy.

As for Kasongo, who adopted Tshakua with me, he's gone for good and we haven't heard any more about him. Except for once. I don't know what got into him, but for some reason or other he wanted to see Tshakua again and rang him up.

"I'll come and collect you for Christmas," he said.

I was delighted and agreed at once. Kasongo was living with a West Indian woman, and Tshakua went to stay with them. But early on in the holidays, before Christmas, Kasongo phoned again.

"I'm going to have to bring back." he said.

"But why? You asked him to stay with you for the holidays!"

"Well, I've got to bring him back! And I'm not likely to ask him again! I wanted to keep in touch with him – that's why I came and fetched him – but he's too badly behaved. I can't keep him."

"Bring him back as soon as you like!" I said. "He's wanted here! I'll be glad to have him back – I didn't ask you to take him!"

I was beside myself!

"I don't even know where you live! I didn't even try to find out your telephone number to tell you what I thought of you when you left us without any money or anywhere to live, and me without a job! If you'd really loved Tshakua you'd at least have had him with you until I could get myself sorted out. And now everything's going well for us, now I have a flat, a job and a husband, have I ever asked you for anything? Did I ring you up and ask you to come and fetch the boy? And now you have the nerve to ring me up and say 'I won't do it again'! What sort of a man are you?"

So he brought Tshakua home. I tried to find out what had happened.

"What did he do?" I asked. "Explain! Have you got any reasons?"

"Yes! I've got some new leather armchairs, and Tshakua was supposed to sleep on a couple of them! And he wetted all over them! And when he was told off he sulked! And he did this, that and the other too..."

"But he's only a child! And you know perfectly well he wets the bed at night – he always has! When he was smaller we bought nappies, but they don't make them his size now, so we just wash the sheets and dry them, and that's that. As for sulking, what do you expect? You used to be his father, you lived with his mother, and now he finds you with another woman, a stranger. Yes, she is a stranger to him! And you told him off in front of her – it's quite natural he should sulk. He hasn't seen you for a long time, and his relationship with you has altered. He used to think of you as his father, remember – you spent a lot of time looking after him. And perhaps you're not so interested in him now."

"It isn't that! I made him welcome, and the girl who's living with me was quite willing for him to come for the holidays. But for some reason or other he took it into his head to start sulking, and..."

But I'd had enough.

"All right! Let this be the last time, then. And don't come asking to have him again, because I won't let you have him!"

And we've never heard from him since.

At first, after Kasongo left, the social workers at the hospital used to make remarks.

"You shouldn't really keep Tshakua away from his father," they said.

I couldn't believe my ears.

"What can I do?" I said. "I know as well as you do that Tshakua needs his father. He loves him! Do you think I'd refuse to let him see him? I wasn't the one that parted them – it was Kasongo who left!"

I picked up a pen.

"Here's my address and telephone number. There's a file on us here, so you know where Kasongo works. If you want to get in touch with him and give him my address... But I know he's got it already. He was the first person I told when I found somewhere to live. I don't know where he lives, but

I rang him at work and said, 'I've just been given somewhere to live, thank God. You're good with your hands – it would be a help if you'd come round and help me settle in.' And he came. So he knows my address and telephone number."

I don't know whether the social worker ever did get in touch with him, but he never contacted me, except that time when he sent Tshakua back almost as soon as he arrived.

But Tshakua knows even Kasongo isn't his real father. You can tell, because he always calls him Uncle. He always called me Mummy right from the start, and I was very glad. But when Tshakua tried to call Kasongo Daddy, he always corrected him and said, "I'm your uncle."

A child always understands when you talk to him like that. So Tshakua called Kasongo Uncle. But he also realized straight away that he didn't have a father.

The poor boy's certainly learned how to adapt himself! Other people can't imagine how difficult it is for an African to leave home and come and live in Europe. Almost as soon as he arrived, Tshakua was put in a room all on his own in the crèche. Back in his own country he'd been surrounded by all his family ever since he was born. He slept with his elder brother on one side and his aunt on the other, and there were people picking him up all the time.

I had to adapt too when I got here: to the food, to a way of life where people shut themselves up and don't have their families round them. And when my friend, the doctor from Bordeaux, rejected me, I suffered horribly. In my country no one is ever abandoned: there is always the family and friends, the love and kindness of everybody. Back home I didn't work, I lived from day to day. I grew up following the same road as my parents without asking myself any questions. In France, when I found myself all alone without a job or a family or the love of anybody, I had to fight to find my own way.

The doctor who got me to leave Africa had been married there, but by the time I met him and he brought me here he'd left his wife long ago and they were already divorced. As he was free I thought I was making sure of security, not just taking a chance. But after scarcely three months we split up, and I was alone in a country I knew nothing about.

It was he who'd given me the idea of leaving home. It was he who'd suggested I should return to France with him. I agreed because I sometimes saw girls who'd been there, and they were lovely and radiant and I thought life must be easy here. White people coming to our country from France always looked well-off and well-dressed. So did our own people, coming back from France. They were careful not to tell the truth: they just boasted of having seen and done and understood everything. So I imagined Europe as quite different from what it really is.

It was winter here when I arrived, and so cold I had to stay indoors all day. I couldn't believe it: was this really Europe?

I was so naïve! I didn't even know there were trees here – my picture of the world was completely fantastic. I imagined Europe as some enormous city that God had sent down ready-made from the sky, without a speck of dust or dirt or even any soil. Because what had fascinated me in all the films I'd seen back home was the tall buildings, the streets full of cars, the elegant men and women in beautiful apartments. I suppose I couldn't have seen enough films, because I imagined that in Europe there was nothing natural at all.

And now I was finding out that there were seasons, and in particular winter.

I lived for three months with the doctor and his children – and their behaviour was awful. The children didn't understand me at all. They were black, and their parents were African, but they'd been born here and thought I was ridiculous. They didn't show me any respect. To make matters worse, I spoke French very badly and was completely ignorant. I couldn't imagine ever adapting to the life here; it was beyond me.

For example, a few days after I arrived I asked them how to roast a chicken: I'd never used the kind of equipment they had in their kitchen. They showed me what to do, and I cooked the chicken and put it on the table. But I didn't know you were supposed to carve it up with a knife and fork, so I just pulled it apart with my hands.

"I'm not eating that!" they all said, and went and shut themselves up in their rooms.

I couldn't guess that sort of thing, any more

than I knew you had to wash your hands after you'd been to the lavatory! I'd led a completely different kind of life, and I was totally disorientated. And they were proud and contemptuous; they hated me and wouldn't do anything to help me. If their father had been at home to explain things and stand up for me it might have been different. But he was always on duty and spent most of his time at the medical school. I wasn't prepared to stand any more of it. We parted.

My children haven't had to go through that kind of experience. They've adapted themselves almost too well, and now they behave as if they'd been born here.

When we left the hotel and came to live in the flat, I had all kinds of difficulties to cope with: paying the rent, getting enough furniture together, buying all the necessary odds and ends. And sometimes, instead of giving them bread and butter and chocolate for their breakfast, I warmed up some rice left over from the evening before.

"Have some rice, darling," I'd say to Tshakua. "There isn't any milk today."

Tshakua stared.

"Mum! I can't have rice for breakfast!"

As if there was something unnatural about it! As if it matters what you eat for breakfast – chocolate or rice or anything else – so long as it's nourishing! Sometimes I really didn't have enough money for milk, and there wasn't anything but rice to eat in the house, but I'd think, "Never mind, as long as there's something!"

But he made things difficult because he'd grown up here and thought like a European.

"Mum – I don't want that! I want my breakfast!"

One day I bought some fish like the fish we have back home. I thought it would be a treat. I was very excited, and called Tshakua into the kitchen to see.

"Look, darling – I'm going to cook some fish the way we do it back home!"

When I dished it up he took the tiniest possible taste.

"It tastes funny! Not like the fish in the canteen. And it smells horrible!"

To me that fish is the best and most delicious food there is, and it's so expensive I can practically never have it: it's imported and costs a fortune. That day, when for once I could afford it, I couldn't wait to get it home: I thought we'd all enjoy it so much, the children and I. They do have smoked fish here too, but in our country they cover it with charcoal and cook it in its own juice till it goes all black. It's delicious. But Tshakua wouldn't eat it because it was funny and not like the fish they served in the canteen!

I know I didn't choose an easy life. With a child who's ill and husbands who didn't understand me, I've had to fight. But I managed on my own. And it was because I did that I managed to get anywhere.

I've always been prepared to put up a fight to make things better for myself. When I was young, back home, and saw someone else succeed at something, I wanted to be like them. If another pupil

MY OWN CHOICE

worked hard at school and came top of the class when I was only third or fourth, I was jealous. I was always comparing myself with other people. In those days I wasn't very religious, but I used to think, "Please, God, tell me how I can get to be like him!"

I had to do it. I didn't have a moment's peace until I felt equal to the people I admired. I know jealousy's wrong, but I can't help it. I need to fight. And when all's said and done, it's stood me in good stead.

I wasn't born in the capital of my own country, or even in a town that had electricity. I was born in a village. My father was a chief there; a customary chief. Then he got a job in a shop in the town. It wasn't a very big town, but it was much bigger than the village: it even had a prison! And schools, and a sort of motel, and electricity in the European quarter. White people had lived there once; there were fine houses in that part of the town, with showers and all sorts of modern conveniences. Some of our own people lived in them now. When we got our independence the Whites all left, but some of the people who'd worked for them as clerks and secretaries got their former bosses' old jobs and went to live in their houses.

But my father lived in the poor part of the town. He sold all kinds of things: matches, sugar, rice, sweets, biscuits, clothes, paraffin... almost anything. After a while he sent for those of his children who wanted to go to school, or rather those who were up to it. They were my half-brothers and half-sisters;

my father had had lots of wives. It was then that I started to learn French, at the state school. And it was there I began to take my studies seriously: I realized I wanted to learn. What helped me see it was that I went to school more regularly than I had in the village, because the school was in the European quarter, which filled my imagination. It was quite near where we lived, too.

Back in the village I'd started school when I was seven. It was a Catholic school and the teachers were priests. They'd been there for years, but instead of teaching in French they now used only the local language because all the settlers had gone. So until I was twelve or thirteen I could only read and write my native language. It's the only one the rest of my family know.

I only went to that first school occasionally because it was so far away. We had to get up at four in the morning and walk for hours. We took something to eat with us on the way – our parents got it ready for us the day before. They mixed rice and gravy together and wrapped it up tight in big leaves that we carried slung over our shoulders. So, laden with our bags and our lunches, we made for a wide river eleven kilometres away. Perhaps it was only eight or ten kilometres, I can't remember exactly now. But I do remember it seemed endless. We used to smarten ourselves up after we'd crossed the river. We put our bags down on the far bank and washed ourselves – splashed ourselves all over. The sun was hot already. We dressed without bothering to dry ourselves: by the time we got to school we were quite dry. And in the evening we had to go all the way back again. It was exhausting. I did it for three or four days, but on the fourth I hadn't the heart. My parents woke me up but I made excuses. Said I was too tired, that my feet hurt.

The town where my father worked was quite small, and when I started thinking things over I realized it didn't suit me. I wanted a change. In our country, girls of fifteen or sixteen start to have breasts and ideas. An uncle of mine – one of my father's younger brothers – worked in a larger town. So off I went, without telling anyone. My uncle used to come and see us sometimes and I'd already asked him if I could go and live with him. He'd promised to make the necessary arrangements. But one day I got the chance to join a group of tourists, so I went with them, without having to buy a ticket.

In my country a girl of that age likes to be well-dressed; she wants people to look at her. I'd realized my father wasn't rich enough to give me the things I dreamed of. When my uncle came, I could see he'd done better for himself. He had a more interesting and eventful life. He was an accountant: he paid out people's salaries, and earned a lot of money himself. My mind had been made up for a long time: I wanted to live with my uncle and go on with my studies.

It was when I was there that I had my baby. I was seventeen or eighteen at the time. The baby's father was married. My uncle's wife was very angry and my pregnancy caused a lot of problems. So I went back to live with my mother, and she helped me bring up the baby. But it was she who looked after him most.

I'd met various people at my uncle's, and when the baby was two or three years old I left him with my mother and went back to the town where my uncle lived. But I didn't like it there any more. I thought it over: I'd been bored in the village; even here I wasn't living the kind of life I wanted. I began to think of going to live in the capital. Some of my father's family lived there, including my aunts. I didn't really know what I was after, but I did know I hadn't got it yet. So I thought I'd go and live with one of my aunts, and I kept my eyes open for an opportunity.

One day I heard that an army plane was flying from the town where I was to the capital, transporting military equipment. So I wangled myself a pass and got on board. I didn't need a ticket; it didn't cost me a penny.

I'd jumped at the opportunity and hadn't had time to tell my aunt I was coming. I didn't quite know what to do when we landed, but I managed somehow to get from the airport to where she lived. She hadn't seen me since I was very small, and I had to introduce myself. She was very surprised to see me, and when I think about it now I'm not sure she was very pleased. All I knew then was that she was my aunt and that I wanted to live in the capital.

And that's where I met the doctor who brought me to Europe.

I'm sure it was God who made me take all those

decisions. I didn't know at the time, myself, what force was driving me on. But I know now. If I'd stayed back in my own country, Tshakua would never have come to France, where he has been treated and cared for.

CHAPTER FOUR

He's got the virus but he isn't ill

Whenever Tshakua goes into hospital I move in too. The nurses are always astonished.

"Why are there two people in here? Are you going to sleep with him?"

"Yes," I answer. "I've always done it. I'm afraid he might need something during the night, or have a temperature, or ring the bell when there's no one there to answer. So I prefer to stay with him."

Some nurses suggest I should sleep in the chair by his bed. But I refuse. I sleep with him. I always sleep near my darling when he's ill or when he's got a temperature. I can tell when the fever's gone down and he feels better, because then he goes and visits other patients or watches the television. I don't mind, then, if they sit me in a chair or whatever. But when he's feverish I always hold him in my arms. Even at home I go and sleep with him if he's been unwell during the night. And then in the morning I take him in to the hospital, by train or in an ambulance, and I move in at the same time as he does.

When they see me in his room in the hospital, they say;

"But Tshakua's a big boy now! He's quite capable of being on his own!"

"No!" I answer. "He's still very young. My son's ill and I won't be separated from him."

The nurses can't stay with him all night. Besides, he asks me to stay.

"You will stay, won't you, Mum?"

"Yes, darling. You go to sleep. I won't leave you."

And later on, he says:

"I feel all right now, Mum. You go home. I'll watch the television."

I always plug in the television before I go: I know that when he feels all right he'll watch it and won't need anyone.

One day Tshakua was at the hospital for the day, as usual. When I can't bring him home myself he's allowed to come by ambulance. I leave him at the hospital in the morning and go to work, then when it's time for him to come home I ring the ambulance man:

"Will you bring Tshakua home now, please?"

Later on I take a minute off work and ring home to make sure he's got back safely.

But that day when I phoned home he wasn't there. Not back by three o'clock? I knew the ambulance man picked him up from the hospital at half-past one, after the children had had their lunch. And he still wasn't home at half-past three! I called the hospital.

HE'S GOT THE VIRUS BUT HE ISN'T ILL

"We kept him in because his temperature suddenly shot up."

"You mean you're taking him in?"

"Yes."

"I'll be there right away."

I'd just been going to start work at a lady's house, but now I put my coat on again.

"I'm afraid I can't stay. My son's been taken ill and I have to go and see what's happening."

I took the metro to the hospital and went up to his room.

"What's wrong, darling?"

"I've got a pain, Mum!"

"It'll soon be better."

I went to see the doctors.

"It's nothing serious," they explained. "We've done a check-up. But it may be the start of an infection. We'll give him an antibiotic."

I began to cry. Whenever he's got a pain or a fever I nearly go out of my mind with anxiety. Perhaps he's going to have diarrhoea? I've been told so often they don't know when the illness might become active! As soon as he feels unwell I panic: I always think they're going to have to tell me the bad news. When they do, if that day ever comes, I don't know how I'll bear it.

They reassured me. What with the antibiotics and the drip and all the other things they'd done, his temperature would soon go down. There was nothing to worry about. I'd missed my morning's work, so I decided to work that evening.

"Darling," I said, "I must go to work now, but

I'll come back and stay with you for the night."

My husband was at work. I called him.

"Tshakua's in hospital, so I won't be coming home. When I leave work at eight or half-past I must come back to the hospital. So I won't be able to have dinner with you."

Then I went to see the sister.

"Is it all right if I come back later on?"

I knew I had to let them know because of security.

Then off I went to my cleaning, without stopping for anything to eat. When I came back, Tshakua was just the same. I took him in my arms and we slept together. By the morning I was very hungry.

I hadn't eaten anything at all the day before. When I should have been having lunch I was trying to find out what had happened to Tshakua. And after that I was too busy rushing to and fro. And now I had to leave him and go to work again. But I was hungry. When the morning shift came on duty and a male nurse appeared, I asked him:

"Could you let me have a piece of bread and a drop of hot milk? I didn't have time to have anything to eat yesterday."

He was very understanding and did as I'd asked.

"Would you like some, darling?" I asked Tshakua.

"Oh no, Mum!"

I was sorry he didn't have any appetite. I forced myself to eat, but I was depressed, I felt queasy, I'd slept badly and I was tired. And as I'd come straight to the hospital the previous evening without calling in at home, I hadn't been able to wash and change.

A West Indian girl who worked in the hospital went by in the corridor. I knew her – I'd often seen her there. I thought she might help me.

"I've been here all night with my son, who's ill, but I haven't got any toilet things with me. If you could let me have a piece of soap and something to dry my face with before I go to work – "

But she started to lecture me.

"Look, this isn't a hotel, you know! People ought to bring their own things with them! You've already asked for bread and I don't know what, and now – "

I was crying by now. I came out into the corridor and shouted at her.

"It's obvious you haven't got any problems! Why do you have to treat me like this? You don't know what it is to be anxious all the time! How was I to know my son was going to have to go into hospital? He was only supposed to come in for the day! Then, when I phoned, they told me he'd got a temperature and they were keeping him in. Was I supposed to go home first for some soap and some bread before I came to see him? God, if you can see this, tell me how such things are possible!"

By now the rest of the staff had stopped to listen to us. There we all were in the corridor – nurses and maids, the West Indian girl, and me wrapped up in my sheet, As I hadn't got a nightdress with me I'd made do with a hospital sheet. I didn't want to crumple my clothes; I had to look presentable to go to work. I felt like an object of pity, standing there in my sheet, asking for a bit of soap, and all she could do was make stupid remarks. I hated her.

"What's happened to me could happen to anybody, you know! Do you think I like coming here instead of going quietly home to my family? And you – instead of trying to help, all you can do is sit in judgment!"

I looked her straight in the eye.

"We never know what might happen, any of us. Today it's my turn. Tomorrow it may be yours!

"I can wait!" she yelled. "I can wait!"

She was lucky enough to be healthy. She had no idea what I was talking about.

"What do you want me to do? Kill myself!"

The others tried to calm me down.

"Come on, you mustn't talk like that!"

"Oh yes, I must! If I understand correctly, I'm here to amuse myself! I came here just for fun, instead of staying at home with my husband and children! But my son's ill! I didn't go home first because I was in a panic. I slept here to be with my son. And this is how she treats me! 'People ought to bring their own things!' If you'd seen the state I was in yesterday!"

She was shouting at the same time as I was, but I didn't listen to her. The nurses separated us. I went and locked myself up in the ladies' room and cried my eyes out. Then I went back to be with my son. I knelt down in his room and prayed. He watched.

HE'S GOT THE VIRUS BUT HE ISN'T ILL

"What are you crying for, Mummy?" he asked.

"Nothing, darling. I always cry when you're ill and people are unkind."

Then I kissed him and went out into the corridor. The West Indian woman was still there.

"Forgive me for speaking to you like that," I said. "I was being a nuisance – I won't do it again. Even if I have to come and sleep here unexpectedly because my son's ill, I'll just get up in the morning, splash my face with water and go. I'm sorry."

She'd calmed down a bit too.

"The thing is, some people really are a pain. They think we haven't got anything to do but run about after them, and..."

But I didn't feel like listening.

"No, it's for me to apologize," I said. "I was the one who started it."

Then I walked away. "It's incredible," I thought. "What a life! You try to bear your burdens as best you can, and people just can't see how difficult it is. How could I simply accept such indifference? We all need other people's support! We need them to be near us, to try to understand us, to love us a little. But it seems that's too much to ask."

It's true I do feel lonely sometimes. My son was ill, and I had to leave him and go to work. I'd have liked to stay and watch him to see if he was getting better, but I had to go because my boss wouldn't understand if I didn't. And on top of it all that girl had to come and scream at me! I felt very hurt. She should have helped me – it was up to her to ask me, "What can I do to help you?"

And instead she'd put me in the wrong.

I'm lost when Tshakua's ill. I get scared. Sometimes I find him just sitting there with his head in his hands. Not playing marbles, not drawing, not even watching television. I rush up to him:

"Darling, what is it?"

"I'm just a bit tired."

At other times he'll be watching television and then suddenly announce:

"Mummy, I'm going to bed."

In broad daylight.

"Have you got a pain?"

"No, I just want to have a little sleep. I'm a bit tired."

When these things happen it's as if there were a hand clutching my heart. "What is it?" I wonder. Has something triggered off the illness? Are all the medicines he's been taking for so long, day and night, making him tired? I feel weighed down.

But when I see him laughing and enjoying himself I'm overjoyed. Now my husband's children are here Tshakua often plays with them in their room. He's bigger than they are and he likes playing school: he's the teacher and gives them homework to do. On Sunday, if it's fine, we all go for a walk in the park, and the children play football. I can relax. I find myself feeling quite hopeful.

When Tshakua looks bright and cheerful in the morning, I try to plan something nice for him that day.

"What do you fancy to eat?"

If he does fancy anything particular, he tells me.

"I'd like a couscous, with meat and chick peas!"

That's his favourite dish.

But sometimes he only says:

"Nothing, Mum – I'm not hungry."

That always frightens me. One day at the hospital I asked the doctors about it.

"He used to eat a lot when he was little, and now he's got hardly any appetite. What's going on?"

They reassured me.

"There's no need to worry – he's growing quite normally. Perhaps it's because the weather's so hot just now. Lots of people aren't very hungry in the summer. They're more likely to be thirsty."

I know I worry too much: I try to check up on him every moment of the day, every detail. As soon as I get up in the morning I have to know how he slept, what woke him up, how he feels. If he says he's got a headache before he goes to school, I'm in despair all day, I can't think of anything else. And it happens often, especially since he had an operation for sinusitis.

I usually stay with him when he's in hospital, but that time I went to work while they were waiting for him to come round from the anaesthetic. The doctors had said the operation wasn't dangerous. But when he woke up there was no one there, and as the tubes were uncomfortable he pulled them out. And they couldn't give him another anaesthetic to put them in again. They told me it didn't matter very much. But now he's always having headaches, and I'm sure that's when it started. The one time I wasn't with him! He hasn't had swollen glands for a long time, but he often has a headache. He hasn't had a temperature, either, since the day I had the row with that woman at the hospital. He's growing up just like other children; in fact he's very tall for his age and very sturdy. And at the moment he's well.

We had much more trouble during his first few years at school, when he was often ill. I used to think, "Perhaps it's all that medicine! He's been taking it for so long – it could easily be a strain on the nerves or the brain."

But I don't want to throw any doubt on his medicine. If I didn't believe in the treatment I wouldn't be so careful about seeing he follows it. I wouldn't bother. As it is, I think about it all the time and make sure he takes his medicine every day.

A couple of months ago, when I'd just had an operation myself, the ambulance man came to pick him up and take him to the hospital for the day. I was too tired to take him myself: there was nowhere for me to lie down while I waited. Usually I took him in, went away and did my shopping, then came back and took him home again. But we had an arrangement by which the ambulance man would take him or bring him home if necessary, and on the day I'm talking about he did both.

I was still lying down when Tshakua came home.

He came and sat down by the bed and I asked him how he'd got on.

"Did everything go all right?"

"Yes."

"Where's the folder?"

He's got a folder where I always keep the notes of his appointments and prescriptions and my own social security card. I give it to him to give to the nurses when he goes to the hospital, and when he gets back I check to see what they've added. I looked in the folder now, but couldn't see the usual note with the date of his next appointment. Strange. I looked again. No, it wasn't there, and there wasn't any prescription either. I felt a kind of dread. Was this a bad omen? As a rule they give him one prescription for DDI and another for Bactrim, and I keep them both on me in case of need.

I knew I still had a small supply of DDI. I like to have some in reserve, and when my husband can call at the hospital pharmacy he collects the main supply. But they wouldn't give it to him without the prescription.

"But what happened, Tshakua? Why didn't they give you another appointment and a prescription?"

I'd rather have asked the ambulance man for an explanation, but he'd just dropped Tshakua at the door and gone off.

"I don't know! The ambulance man came to collect me, we went into the nurses' office as usual, and they gave us back the folder and told us to go."

"Told you to go? Without another appointment and without any DDI prescription? Does that mean you're not ill any more?"

I wasn't too worried about the Bactrim: they might just have decided to drop it. But the DDI! I jumped off the bed, grabbed my phone card, rushed down to the phone box and called the ambulance man. He wasn't home yet, so I called the hospital.

"Did you see my son today?" I asked.

"Yes."

"Well, what's going on? Don't you want him to come and see you any more?"

"Of course we want him to come!"

"Then why isn't there anything in his folder? No date for another appointment, not even a prescription for DDI!"

They were in a panic. One nurse said she didn't know anything about it, another that it wasn't anything to do with her, a third said something else... I lost my temper.

"Don't you take it seriously? Playing about with the life of my son! For once I can't come with him because I'm ill myself, and you let him come home without anything in his folder! What if I hadn't been here, or hadn't bothered to check?"

They went to fetch the doctor.

"I'm sorry about this," he said. "The doctor who used to see him has left. I'm new here and didn't know what the arrangement was."

"If you don't know what you're supposed to do then I'm sorry. You're not doing your job properly! You're playing with his life!"

I was so furious I started saying the first thing that came into my head.

"What am I supposed to do now? It can't wait – I haven't even got enough DDI to be going on with!"

"Can't you send someone?"

"No, I can't send someone! Everybody else is at work, and I'm ill!"

He apologized, the nurses apologized, and the more they all apologized the angrier I got. I couldn't calm myself.

"Right, then! Get everything ready. Ill or not, I'll come and get the date for the next appointment myself! And I'll collect the DDI as well while I'm about it!"

I don't treat his medicine lightly. I think it might give him headaches or weaken his nerves. If he's been naughty, or done badly at school, he gets very anxious and upset. Even I, at my age, would have had enough of the stuff after six months! And he's been taking it all his life, ever since he was a tiny baby. I'm a Christian, I say my prayers, and I've always asked God, "Lord, why has my son got to take all this medicine? I know it's thanks to You that he's in good health, but please help the scientists find the miracle cure that will save him." That's the only thing I wish for.

When I went to the hospital myself, recently, to talk to them about having an operation on my Fallopian tubes, I wept when I thought about Tshakua: "What if I die? What sort of a life would he have? I've been mother and father both to him – I've watched over him right from the start... If only I don't die before he does! I don't know what would become of him if I did! He might be placed with a family where they reject him. They might be frightened of him, like Manga. At any rate, they could never give him what I've given him!"

So I was miserable, and didn't want to have the operation. I was thinking of him, not myself. Anyhow, I've decided not to have it done yet. I'll wait for a bit. The doctors have said there's no hurry: it's up to me to say when I want it done. I had one operation last year, and another a couple of months ago, and the symptoms could recur. I asked the doctor why I was never quite right in spite of all these operations, and he did a drawing to explain. I've got some germ that was there for a long time without being properly treated, and that's what makes my tubes swell. Every time I have an operation they take away the bit that hurts, but it comes back again. I'm supposed to take great care of myself, and in theory to get plenty of rest. And the treatment may do the trick. But the trouble could come back. I don't know what I ought to do, because I have to be able to take care of Tshakua.

It's hard on a mother to have to ask herself this sort of question, but perhaps it's because of it that I love him so. When I tried to have another child I couldn't. Yet I really did want that baby. And to console myself I thought that perhaps I'd lavished on Tshakua all the love I'm capable of giving a child. What I dread is finding myself left with nothing. The doctors won't make any promises. They've told me often I may lose him one day.

I don't know why they want me to keep on

worrying: his health is quite good now. He still takes his medicine, but he doesn't need to hide any more, because all the family now know. And so long as he's happy, that's all I ask. And he has got everything here to make him happy now, with all of us around him – his mother and father and his little brothers and sisters. He never asks any more if he can go and play at someone else's place. And I don't have to say no any more. The days go by peacefully, and I'm content, because all I want is to make him forget his suffering.

Before, he often used to ask:

"Mum, why do I have to go on taking medicine?"

And I would answer:

"Because you're ill."

And then I'd say:

"But it'll all be over one day."

He's been in good spirits ever since my husband's children have been here. The weather's getting better now too: they'll soon be able to go out and play on their bikes. He loves playing; he loves life. He's always doing something. In the hospital he goes around and chats to the other patients in their rooms. He's a child who loves life.

Yesterday there was a ring at the door, and it was some little boys who live in this building, going round asking all the parents to sign a petition for a basketball court. They're going to hand it in at the town hall. Tshakua was so pleased!

"We're going to have a basketball court, Mum! I'll go and play all the time – every Wednesday, every weekend! And Uncle Ngenda's promised to put me down for football..."

He's such a cheerful child. He was eleven in July, and he really does enjoy life. The school has sent for me several times because they say he's too rowdy.

"He can be a bit rough when he's playing, and sometimes he hurts the other boys."

He doesn't like being on his own. He gets bored and depressed. But as soon he's with his friends he's happy: he plays, he runs about, he needs to work off his energy. Sometimes he gets into fights. But he's growing up like all the other children. He's fine.

It's only at school that things aren't all they might be. He loved going when he was small, but he was away ill so often then that he couldn't keep up. So his friends kept going up a class and leaving him behind. I think that's where the trouble started. And maybe all that medicine made it difficult for him to concentrate.

In the end they decided he was too big to stay among the little ones. It's true he's very tall. He takes the same size shoes as I do. Size six. So they sent him on a special course to get him ready for secondary school. But I worry because he meets a lot of young louts there. It's the sort of place that caters mostly for problem children. Some of them are under the psychologist. His teacher often sends for me to complain that he doesn't work and won't be corrected. And as I don't want to tell her all about his problems, she can't really understand. It's a worry.

He's been at this place for three years now. The other children move on, but he's still there. He's had the same teacher for three years, and they can't stand the sight of one another.

"Your son doesn't do any work," she says. "And he won't listen to a word I say."

I know. He's tired of seeing the same person again every morning. Fortunately they've decided at last that he's to move on to secondary school. He's not quite up to it, but he's too big to stay where he is. I hope he'll do better in future. He has been working harder since he heard he's going on to the other school. The headmistress sent for me and told me his marks were improving, and his teacher confirmed it.

I've noticed it too. I give him little tests to see if he's making progress. For instance, on Sunday, when we go in to Paris to church, I let him lead the way.

On the train and in the metro he has to tell us when to get on and off, so I can tell he can read the names of the stations. The same thing on the way back. Sometimes I send him shopping. I dictate a list before he goes: at first that was rather difficult, but now he manages quite well. I give him the money, and he brings back the check-out ticket and the change. He gets just what I've told him to and gives me the right change. He's adjusted well, and I'm very pleased and proud.

I'm not so pleased when he starts asking questions about why he has to take medicine and other children don't. I explain as best I can, and point out he's not the only one. There's Ngado, a little Rwandan boy he meets at the hospital, and Mateso, a little Congolese girl. There are others too.

I always tell him things will be better one day. I want to set his mind at rest as far as possible. After all, the doctor says that even if he's HIV-positive he's not ill yet! And I know he's not infectious, I've been told it's not dangerous to live with him, and I understand. But not everybody does. The men who lived with me and thought it was dangerous – they left! And the other children, at school: no one's ever explained anything to them, so how could they understand? And then there was the time I sent him round to play at a neighbour's house, and they found his AZT... They thought AZT meant the person who had it had AIDS, and they closed their door to him!

Of course I know he might have done something wrong. But only one of the little things all children do. At home, for instance, it doesn't matter how much I keep on at him I can't get him to clean his teeth. He's got holes in some of them, but he just won't brush them. Nor his hair, for that matter. But I'm only talking about little things – the kind of silly tricks all kids get up to. He plays with little girls too, but they don't get up to anything – nothing that matters. And everyone knows that when children go to somebody else's place they may nick a toy or something. Nobody takes any notice.

I'm not strict enough with him. I do punish him sometimes, though. I know what he likes, and

HE'S GOT THE VIRUS BUT HE ISN'T ILL

I try to deprive him of it. For example, I know he loves watching television: he wouldn't mind if you left him in front of it all day. So sometimes I say:

"Tshakua, you've done such and such a thing, and as a punishment I shan't let you watch television today. Go to your room."

"All right, Mum."

But afterwards I know he must be sad, so I have to go and bring him back. I go to his room, and there he is, sitting with his elbows on his knees and his head between his fists. So I give in. I always give in. I can't bear to see him sad. I go over and stroke his cheek and say:

"Don't you feel well?"

"I'm all right, Mum."

"What's the matter then?"

"I'm tired."

"Never mind – come with me. You can watch television if you like."

I give in. Perhaps I shouldn't.

I was stricter with Pierre. I didn't have any trouble with him when he was small, but later on he started smoking and mixing with rougher kids, and I put my foot down.

"Do you really think you're entitled to smoke, at your age, without any money and without a job?"

I was really cross. He was only fifteen – much too young to start to smoke! And we weren't that rich! There he was, still at school – was I supposed to buy him cigarettes instead of food? I was very firm with him.

Pierre was naughty sometimes when he was

small, though not as often as Tshakua. But I was more indulgent with Tshakua because he was ill. Everybody tells me:

"You make his illness an excuse for spoiling him."

He must know I can't bring myself to scold or punish him. If I did I'd feel as if I was hurting someone who'd been hurt already. He takes advantage of it. I used to punish Pierre when he was naughty, and he was frightened of me. But Tshakua isn't a bit afraid of me. He knows I need to see him happy. Otherwise I start thinking he must be ill, and then I'm so scared I can hardly breathe. I don't think I could ever be really harsh with him.

The men who lived with me often tried to change me.

"You won't always be able to be with him. Later on he'll have to manage for himself. You shouldn't let him get away with everything! You're not doing the best for his future. We all love our children, but it's wrong to go too far. You should learn to be firm with him, and treat him just the same as the others."

But I can't do it. I've seen him suffer so much! I've been so afraid for him! I tell myself: all right, let him stay as he is – it's too bad if he has some faults, I'm not going to try to change him. I've loved him as he is; other people can do the same.

And I shall always be with him. Always. I pray to God to preserve me so that I can always be by his side, even when he's grown-up, even when he's married and has a family of his own. His wife may take my place some day, but I hope he'll still need me for some things. I hope that for some things I'll always be irreplaceable. Anyway, I almost never leave him. I have sometimes sent him to my brother's for the holidays, but, what with one thing and another, it's seldom possible for us to be separated. Even in the ordinary way I take my telephone card to work with me, and often ring up to make sure he's all right.

When he's tired all my own strength ebbs away – life doesn't mean anything any more. And when he won't eat, I'm not hungry either: I can't bring myself to touch anything.

I've become so attached to him. Even my own child, back in my own country, doesn't affect me as deeply as he does. Of course I love the other child: I carried him for nine months. But apart from giving birth to him I haven't done much for him. Whereas I adopted Tshakua as soon as I first set eyes on him, and looking after him has made me come to feel like his mother; I am his mother. I've wept for him, I've been afraid for him, I've given him his medicine in secret a thousand times, I've slept in his warmth, I've shared his fever. He's my little boy.

He really is little. He still wets the bed. I know it's psychological and that it'll stop when he's older. I wetted the bed for a long time myself. But I do try to help him break the habit. Sometimes, when I say, "Tshakua, if you don't wet the bed tonight I'll give you this, that or the other," the sheets are quite dry in the morning. The problem is definitely in his head. So the other day, as he'd been sleeping in a bunk bed above one of my husband's sons, I said:

"If you manage not to wet the bed at all until your birthday, you shall have a bed of your own as a present."

And he did manage it for several nights. As soon as I saw the battle was won I went and bought the bed, complete with mattress, and even some sheets and a pillow-case so that he should have everything new. He was wild with joy at having his own bed in his own little corner. I pressed my advantage:

"If you keep it up you can have your own desk. You're going to secondary school, so you shall have your own desk, instead of having to work with your brothers and sisters. And your own wardrobe and everything."

He was so pleased! He's made a great effort and had only one accident in ten days. That was last night. But now I'm sure the problem will soon be solved.

I myself have never been able to bring myself to tell Tshakua that he's HIV-positive. How could I do such a thing? But the doctors will make a start. They work with the psychologists, and psychologists know a lot about children – they'll be able to make him understand. I'd rather he learned the truth from a psychologist. He'll be better at explaining things to him gradually.

I don't see how *I* could just blurt out:

"You know, darling, you're ill. You're HIV-positive."

He'd ask me what it meant, and I wouldn't know what to say. I don't want to tell him it can lead to AIDS. He watches television, he hears people talking, he knows all about it! He knows AIDS can kill someone in the end. I couldn't let the words cross my lips. I've always told him his illness is one that lasts a long time but that it will end some day.

So I'm quite willing for the doctor or the psychologist to talk to him. He's getting older, and when he's fifteen or sixteen he'll start going out with girls, and that might cause some problems. So let them tell him about all that.

But I don't want people telling him he's ill. He's not ill. He just has to be watched over, protected, taken care of, loved, given the sort of things all children need. He's a bearer of the virus, but he isn't ill.

They've told me the virus could trigger off AIDS quite suddenly. I've asked them about it a hundred times. They say Tshakua may go on as he is for a long time, but it's also possible the disease could appear out of the blue. May God spare me! Perhaps, at the beginning, I might have been able to get over it. But now I know I never could.

But it's not going to happen. We've not won yet, but I have a feeling my son is going to grow up. I'm sure of it. I trust in God. I pray all the time. And I know there is a God. Whenever I have worries or troubles, I pray and fast. I don't bother about anything else, I just weep and say, "God, please help me! I leave the problem in your hands. Please help me!"

I like to know what's going on. I often talk to the doctors. Whenever I take Tshakua to the hospital I ask for explanations if I get the chance. I want to know everything. Why they stopped the AZT; why they're only giving him DDI. It seems DDI is a new drug that's more efficient than AZT. I want to understand everything, especially when they interrupt the treatment, because sometimes they suspend it for a month or a fortnight.

"Why have you stopped the treatment?"

"Why have you started the treatment up again?"

They say:

"We've stopped the treatment because the blood-count's down. We can't start it up again until the number of globules increases. The drug we're giving him is very powerful and we don't want him to have too much of it. So we check up once a fortnight to see what's happening to the globules."

They explain it all to me. They're very kind. The social worker's kind too; she's a great help to me. It does me good to talk to someone who can give me some moral support. She's given me a lot of advice. But I don't need anyone now; I decide things for myself. Once she asked me how Tshakua was getting on at school. I admitted:

"He's been ill so often he's got rather behind, and he doesn't work as hard as he should."

She suggested sending him as a boarder to a place in Paris where they deal with children with problems.

"The pupils there are monitored by psychologists, but at the same time it's an ordinary school. And they'd make sure he kept up with his treatment. I think it would be a very good thing for him.

HE'S GOT THE VIRUS BUT HE ISN'T ILL

You could go and see him there and have him home at the weekend. Think it over, and if you're interested we'll make an application."

I was in favour, except about letting him be a boarder.

"All right," I said, "but I want to take him there in the morning and bring him back in the evening. I want him to sleep at home. A week is too long to go without seeing him."

I need to see him every evening, to watch him moving about, to know if he's all right, to know if he's happy. I love him too much to wait for the weekend – I'd feel as if I'd stopped breathing. I don't know why I love him so. It's a terrible love. Perhaps it comes from all the sleepless nights I've spent worrying about him, from all the suffering I've accepted for his sake, from all we've shared.

Who would notice, at boarding school, if his temperature suddenly shot up during the night and he started to shiver? And who'd do anything about it? No, I have to be with him. Whenever he's feverish I soak a towel in cold water and put it on his forehead. I'm ill when he's ill; if he's in pain, I hurt all over. When I hear him laugh my heart is light; when he looks unhappy it thumps like a sledgehammer. How could I part with him? I don't trust anybody else to look after him properly. I'd be too frightened.

The social worker told me to go and talk to her if I had any problems. I go to see her nearly every Wednesday. I see the doctors too, and the nurses. We work as a team. Everyone rallies round for

Tshakua's sake; everyone loves him. Sometimes the nurses say, "How he's changed!" when he comes in.

Some of them who've known him since he was a year old are still there. One will give him a kiss, another will put her arm round his neck and say:

"He's grown even more since last time! He's taller than I am now!"

It's true. My son's very tall and well-built. Handsome and really sturdy. A good-looking boy, with wonderful eyes. He's only eleven, but looks at least twelve or thirteen. And he's so sweet! He loves to be helpful, and I've never heard him say an unkind word to anyone. With me especially he's always very affectionate; I can see he loves me.

Sometimes I talk to him about what he wants to be when he grows up.

One day he said he wanted to be a fireman.

"But they earn hardly anything!" I said.

That didn't worry him in the least.

"But it's only right to help people, Mum! If no one came to get them out when their house is on fire, they'd die! I'd like to be a fireman."

Then he started to tell me about his other plans.

"When I'm grown-up I'll go out to work and you won't have to go out cleaning any more. You'll be able to stay at home and rest."

He's a really sensitive child, and he loves everybody. Even when he was still very small, if anyone gave him anything he'd save it up to share with somebody else. And he's still the same: when he goes to the hospital I always buy him some cakes for after his tests, but he doesn't eat them straight away.

"I won't take them out of the bag till Ngado comes. Then I'll share them with him."

Ngado is a little Rwandan boy. He's HIV-positive too and they met as out-patients at the hospital. I've met his parents. At first they didn't want to talk, but I said:

"There's no point in trying to pretend to each other. We're all in the same boat. The fact that we're here makes that clear enough. There aren't many people we can tell the truth to and talk to about the children's future. So..."

So we became friends. We often ring one another up. Every other Wednesday the children meet at the hospital, and while they're being seen to I talk to Ngado's parents.

"How did he get it?" was the first question.

Their answer was the same as mine. Their son too was born with it.

Something or other had happened to the mother back in Rwanda and she'd had to have a transfusion. The father had come to France already, leaving the mother to have the baby there. When he'd found a job and somewhere to live, he sent the tickets for his wife and family to join him. He didn't know she was HIV-positive – she didn't know herself – and they started living together again. Then one day young Ngado came down with an attack of malaria. The school took him to the hospital, and the hospital did some tests. Then one day they sent for the parents and said:

"Your little boy's HIV-positive."

"Impossible!"

"You'll have to be tested too."

So they were, and they found that the mother was HIV-positive and the father was all right. Life's very complicated. But it's a difficult situation for a man to accept, and their marriage is going through a crisis. He doesn't trust his wife now, and isn't easy in his mind about having relations with her.

One day recently he came to the hospital without her and confided in me.

"It's almost impossible now for us to get along. I brought her to France so that I could take care of the children, but now the whole situation's changed. As far as I'm concerned she can go wherever she likes! I've got the children with me, and that's all I care about."

If I understood him rightly they keep on quarrelling, she runs off to her family, and they just can't get on together any more. I know how difficult it is. I remember. There has to be an understanding like the one I have now with my husband, with each one trying to see the other's point of view. She's the one who's infected, and she ought to realize her husband can't have any idea what she feels. And he ought to realize it's not her fault: she's ill and probably needs to share her troubles with him.

But when will the doctors find a successful treatment? It's urgent. I'm not just thinking of Tshakua. It's urgent for everyone. Here in Europe there are people, children and grown-ups alike, who are still alive because treatment's available to them. But people ought to see what's happening in other countries! When I was in Rwanda I wept my heart out over it. I went back again recently, just before I started this book. And I'm going to ask AIDES what can be done to help the children in my own country.

Sometimes, when I take Tshakua to the hospital, I go up to the wards. And when I look through a door and see someone who's very ill, it pains me so much that I weep. That's all I can do – weep. And, because I'm a believer, pray. That's what I did back home. but I was terribly depressed: I saw more suffering then than I'd ever seen in my life! It's too much! There's not even an aspirin for a child who's got a temperature. Nothing's done there for an HIV-positive child who might be saved here. It's unbearable. I felt desperate. It seemed to me the world was destroying itself. There are thousands of children like Tshakua out there, and they're just dying. Dying because there's not even a drip available, not even an aspirin. Nothing. I was shocked.

A mother with a baby in her arms can see he's got a temperature and can hear how hard it is for him to breathe, but nothing can be done about it. The Europeans ought to try to do something! Perhaps that baby could have been helped if he lived here, because here the authorities do all they can. But out there in the developing countries, what can a mother do?

I could die today, but I'm forty now and have lived. Our children must be given a chance to live before they die! If Tshakua had been a grown-up I wouldn't have done all I have done for him. Of course I'd have been very sorry that my sister's child was ill. I'd have gone to see him; I'd have asked after him; but I wouldn't have got involved the way I did. The reason why he affected me so deeply was that he was a child. He hadn't done anything to deserve what was happening to him. How much time did he have to live before he fell ill? None! He was born ill! And it's for children like that I want to fight. If I can do anything to help protect those poor children out there, I'll do it. I'll organize something myself, with my own small resources, my own energy. I've been able to do something for Tshakua, so why shouldn't I try to do something for the others? I can't not do it; I feel so sorry for them. Even if I can only save ten or twenty of them, I'm going to try.

I want to go out there. And at least take them some AZT or even the most basic drugs. I hope AIDES will be able to help me. I mean to try to save the children of Africa, the children in my own country, the country where I was born and where I lived as a little girl. I know there are children like that everywhere, but I can't forget what I saw out there. It was unbearable.

"But can't you even put them on a drip?" I asked the doctors.

"How can we?" they said. "The hospital hasn't got the necessary materials."

Anyone with the money can go and buy those materials at the chemist's. But the hospital hasn't got anything. I was furious.

HE'S GOT THE VIRUS BUT HE ISN'T ILL

"How did things get into this state? What's the Government doing?"

"The Government!" said the doctors. "That's you. If you can do something about it, go ahead!"

Apparently it would be useless even if you were to get whole truckloads sent there. Everything would get stolen: the doctors would use the drugs in their own surgeries for their own patients, and there'd be none left for the people in hospital. But that's so unfair on the children! They're born, they suffer, and they die, and that's all the life they've had! Why? What have they done? The scientists must forge ahead! People here don't truly realize the extent of the suffering, because here there's all that's necessary for looking after the sick. You have to go to the developing countries themselves to see how dreadful the situation is. Some children there are valued less than a dog would be in Europe.

Myself, I pray to God to perform some miracles. He's already performed one for my son: it was He who arranged that his mother should come to France; that the illness should declare itself here; that despite the death of his mother and the absence of his father there should be someone to look after him; and that he should be in a place where he can be properly looked after. If he'd stayed in Rwanda he'd have been dead and buried long ago; no one would have been able to save him. There wouldn't have been any drugs to give him, and he wouldn't have had enough to eat even though he was ill. And who would have seen that he had antibodies? No one would even have known he was HIV-positive! Tshakua is a child entrusted to me by God.

He has been lucky – he came here. But what about the others? They can't all come to Europe. But all the medicine we need exists here – boxes and boxes, whole crates and truckloads of it. I don't know how I'll manage it yet, but when I'm ready I want someone to come out there with me just to see what it's like. I'll talk to the people at AIDES about it, and start an association.

I wrote this book in order to talk about my son and to get other people interested. I want to persuade them to give a chance to other youngsters in the same situation as his. They must join me in trying to help these poor children: they've lost their mothers and fathers, they're in the most terrible trouble, and yet they're rejected everywhere.

Even here they're rejected, the same as in Africa.

I wonder if Tshakua will forgive me for telling all this. I've written things in this book that I've never dared tell anyone. I've lied and lied to everybody, I've tried to keep it secret. TF1, the television people, wrote to ask if they could come and interview me. I refused. They said I needn't worry, they'd arrange it so that the audience wouldn't see me or know who I was. I decided I'd rather write a book.

Even so it's very painful to display my own child in public – a real child who's close to me, and who's ill without anyone knowing it. I'm telling the story of his life, his illness, and I pay for it with my own anguish.

"You think you can bear anything," my husband said once, "but you can't. That's why you're always ill – and you're going to have to have another operation. You've suffered enough already, yet you want to expose yourself more."

"I know. But I want Tshakua and the others to be able to lead a normal life. I want the answer to be found, I want the doctors to find the medicine everyone's waiting for!"

That's why I'm putting up a fight. I'm doing it for my Tshakua. And if someone came and told me today they'd found a drug that might do him good in the United States, I'd sell everything I have and go there this very day without a moment's hesitation. I'd find courage for anything for his sake. My strength comes to me from him.

I've managed to protect him, and he hasn't had to go back home, because as soon as I saw him all alone in his room in the crèche, as soon as I heard him shout "Mummy!" when I was leaving, I was drawn to him, hooked. Could I shut my eyes now, back home, to a child in the same distress as Tshakua was, a child doomed to die, who perhaps has died since I came back to France? No, I wanted to bring him back with me. But they wouldn't let me.

"Oh no, that's impossible. You'd have to apply to adopt him, and so on and so forth."

Red tape, while the child is dying!

It's to deal with that kind of situation that I want to start an association. I want to encourage people to give children like this a chance to grow up. Even if they're going to die when they're five years old, at least let them be happy till then. And if they must die when they're only two, at least let them enjoy life and be loved and looked after for those two years. These children nobody cares about.

But it isn't even indifference they suffer; it's worse. Everyone actually runs away from such children. Even here, in France, if any of the people I know had found out Tshakua was ill they wouldn't have come near him! I saw what happened with Antoinette and her husband. Even in France, even now, if I hadn't a husband or a home I could leave my son with Sylvie, but if she saw him taking AZT she wouldn't want to have him any more. She'd be too frightened. That's what makes people conceal the truth. The others all think the illness is some kind of a curse that heralds the end of the world. Some of them even say God in his wrath has sent it to punish us for our sins. I've sometimes heard stupid things like that even in church. So I can't tell anyone about Tshakua.

He isn't a child any more. I've brought him that far. I can have a serious discussion with him. I'm so proud. And when I look at him I think that if he'd stayed back home he wouldn't be here any more, he'd have been dead long ago. He mightn't even have lived to be three years old! His father died back home, soon after his mother. So what would have become of the baby there all alone?

And there are thousands of children like that. Like him.

CHAPTER FIVE

He's my child, entrusted to me by God

I've realized God exists and I often fast. Sometimes I fast for three days running: Friday, Saturday and Sunday. I feel I need to. The strange thing is I've usually got a good appetite, and if for any other reason I don't eat I can't leave the house, I get too faint. But when I know I'm fasting for God I don't even feel hungry; not eating doesn't produce the slightest ill-effect.

Our religion requires us to fast. The minister told us so. The children of Israel used to fast once a year, but if we're sad or worried about something we're allowed to fast whenever we like. Our religion says that whenever you're unhappy or anxious you can speak to God or shed your tears before him, and you don't need any intermediary. So that's what I do: whenever I feel the need I fast and pray and weep. I stay at home and lie on the floor and weep. And I know I'm right.

I've had to go and have some tests done because for the last three or four months, I don't know why, I haven't been able to bend down. When

I do bend down it's very painful. I asked the doctor what it was.

He said they couldn't make it out: the results of the tests were normal. But maybe something has started, because I don't really feel well. I've always had problems of some sort, but never anything like this. It's as if something had suddenly collapsed. And now I'm not supposed to work. I've got a doctor's certificate. At first I was off for three weeks; now for another three.

It isn't easy. My husband's got a job but he works only five hours a day and gets only two thousand six hundred francs a month. He works as a cleaner. He's really a builder, but the only job he could find was cleaning. He got more when he was on the dole. He really did all he could to find work, but it wasn't any good. He's done temporary work as a mason, an electrician, all sorts of things: he can do anything. But he couldn't find anything in his own line, so he took the first job he was offered.

And as I haven't got any private insurance... You don't realize until things go really wrong that you need private insurance as well as the social security. Whenever anyone suggested it I always said, "Oh no, I've got the social security – that's enough." But the social security pays next to nothing!

And I've got children to feed, including my husband's three. The social service people say they ought to go back home to Africa because they're here illegally. They haven't got the proper family status. And one of them's got bowel trouble and has to have a special diet. And I've got all three of them living here, as well as Tshakua. (Pierre has gone.) It's difficult.

But I'm not going to let a little thing like that get me down. The worst is over. I've got everything now – a home, a husband, a life! It wouldn't take much to make me perfectly happy. I never get discouraged. Life goes on. There are bad times, I know, but then it all gets sorted out. I'm not going to give up the fight.

On the contrary. I said I was going to start an organization, and I've been working at it. It's called SAVE US. I took advantage of being off work and went to the town hall.

"I want to start an organization to fight against AIDS," I said.

"You'll have to go to the Prefecture for that," they told me.

The woman at the Prefecture was just going home.

"What do you want to start an organization for?" she asked.

"There are children suffering and there's no medicine to give them. Even in the capital, the biggest town in the country! The children were lying on the floor! In the hospital in the capital! And there isn't any medicine. People with money can buy medicine and drips, but what about those who haven't got any money? I cried and cried! Tiny children! What have they done to have to live like that? If I could I'd try to help grown-ups too, but to start with I want to do something for the children.

It's so unfair; it's unbearable. In my own country, the country where I was born! It's horrible."

The woman listened. She'd forgotten about going home.

"You'll have to fill in a form," she said, "and give the organization a name."

"'SAVE US'," I said.

You had to give the names of three people to start an association. I put down my own and my husband's names, and the name of someone I know who lives near us.

"You have to decide how much money the members have to contribute."

"A hundred francs."

She gave me the telephones numbers of organizations that existed already, so that I could go and see them to exchange ideas and addresses.

The third member of our group is a friend of mine, a fellow-countryman. He's interested in the AIDS problem and has many of the same ideas about it as I do: he often goes back there and knows what things are like.

"We have to do something about it," he said. "We could collect old clothes and sell them in the flea-market. And we could ask people for unused medicines and find a way to send them out there."

We need to have a member of the association out there to supervise things on the spot. One of us could go, but we're also looking for someone suitable out there. We haven't had any meetings yet. We're getting the addresses of organizations with aims similar to our own, to see if we can work

HE'S MY CHILD, ENTRUSTED TO ME BY GOD

together. I'm going to see the AIDES people too. And we're going to arrange to go over and see what can be done.

I can spend time on it now because Tshakua has changed lately. Ever since my husband and I have been together I've noticed that Tshakua has altered. He's found a father. I've always thought that's what he was missing: the love of a father.

His father used to be Kasongo. He loved Kasongo very much. And I could see that none of the men I knew after Kasongo had the same relationship with Tshakua as he had. But Tshakua's found that relationship again now, and that's what's helped him so much.

My husband is very good with the children. He can't bring up his own properly and just let Tshakua do as he likes. There are the same rules for everyone. And Tshakua has changed. Even his teacher agrees he's made great progress. The idea of going on to secondary school has acted as a stimulus. I'm glad about it too. In the evening we make him do a bit of extra work in preparation. He brought me some forms to fill in about his grant.

"The money from the grant will be for you, Tshakua," I told him. "You'll be able to choose what you want to buy with it."

He's happy. He's growing fast. He takes size seven in shoes now: a child of eleven! But he looks fourteen or fifteen.

But some of the doctors and psychologists keep pestering me.

"You ought to tell Tshakua the truth! When he

gets to be fifteen he'll start going out with girls – he can't be left in ignorance. He must start to learn the truth: that his mother is dead, to begin with..."

But my husband backs me up.

"No, you shouldn't tell him! Leave him alone. He'll find out. When he's old enough he'll find out for himself. What's the point in giving a child such a shock? Do they want you to hurt him now, after you've been protecting him ever since he was eight months old? If you could you'd have told him from the beginning. How can you go to him now and say, 'I'm not your mother!'?"

Yes, how could I tell him a thing like that? He's sure I'm his mother. How could he doubt it? I've shown him photographs and told him things to make him think so.

"... and then I had to go to work so I put you in the crèche..."

So I've deceived him. That's what makes it difficult. When he was looking at the snaps that were taken in the crèche he asked:

"How did you feed me, then?"

I lied to him.

"I breast-fed you for a while, but I had to stop when I left you in the crèche."

When I saw he was puzzled I wanted to reassure him, so I invented details – how I fed him and for how long, and so on.

But it's the psychologists and doctors and social workers at the hospital who worry me most. He's started to act the silly way all adolescents do, and they say he's growing up and now's the time to talk to him. They tell me to tell him the truth because he knows it already. And it's true they've still got his mother's file at the hospital, and sometimes, when he's waiting in his room for them to examine him, the doctors discuss her case in front of him. And he hears them say:

"His mother, Madame B., died in such and such a year…"

I know that. I'm not always there, but one day I called one of the doctors out into the corridor and said:

"Do you know what you're doing? You're traumatizing that child."

That was two or three years ago. I'd left him there as usual, and gone back to pick him up. There was a group of doctors round him in his room; the ones I knew and some others. And the old ones were telling the others:

"This little boy's mother died in this hospital…"

And Tshakua was there, looking at them.

So I'm quite willing to believe he may know, but he doesn't show it, he doesn't ask me about it. So how could I reveal a thing like that, point-blank, without his asking me? And he never has asked me!

They say:

"He knows but he doesn't like to talk to you about it. It's up to you to take the initiative."

Maybe. But I can't. I haven't got the heart. I could never give my darling Tshakua such a shock. It would be the same as if someone suddenly came and said to me, 'Tshakua can't live with you any more.' Well, I'd never let anyone take him away from me. And I'm not going to take his mother away from him: 'Tshakua, you haven't got a mother. I'm not your mother at all.' If ever he wants to find out for himself, he only has to ask me.

I know what I'll answer.

"If you don't think I'm your mother, all right. But if you're really sure I am your mother, you must just accept it without bothering about anything else. That's all. You're the one who knows whether I'm your mother or not..."

But I'm not going to say anything before he asks.

"...I know I'm your mother," I'll go on. "If anyone's told you otherwise and you agree with them, so be it! But if you know in your heart I am your mother, never mind what they say. And that's all there is to it."

Today I told my husband how I felt when I used to go to the crèche, It would be time to go, but I knew Tshakua would start to cry as soon as I left him there alone in his cot. And so he did! I used to hide outside the door, waiting for him to stop crying. But he didn't. So I used to go in and pick him up.

"Don't cry, my darling, don't cry!"

And I'd try to soothe him. But it was late. I gritted my teeth and prepared to go. But I knew I'd start crying myself when I got out in the corridor. And I'd go on crying all the way to wherever I was going.

I knew from the start he needed me to be his mother. Whenever he called out for someone in the crèche it was me he asked for. The nurses used

HE'S MY CHILD, ENTRUSTED TO ME BY GOD

to take care of him, but it didn't mean anything to him – he could tell it wasn't his mother.

The doctors tried to warn me.

"You must think about it very seriously! You may come to regret the decision you've just made? You know Tshakua's infected..."

And so on. But I wouldn't budge.

"Yes, I know, but I'm prepared to accept all that. Tshakua is my own child. If his mother should get better, we'll share him. That doesn't bother me,"

But as they weren't sure my sister would get better, I felt he was already getting to be my son. So I don't see how I could say to him now:

"You know, Tshakua, you're not really my son."

No, never! And I can't imagine anyone else, Tshakua or anybody, coming and telling me he isn't.

They keep saying he knows anyway. Knows that he had a real mother and that she died in the same hospital he goes to. And they want me to explain to him that someone can have a child without carrying it in her womb.

I know it wouldn't change anything at all for him even if I did tell him the truth, but I can't help being afraid. My husband tries to reassure me that I'm doing the right thing:

"There's no point in telling him."

My brother agrees.

"Let him be. It would only upset him."

I always took more care of Tshakua than of the men who lived with me.

It's only natural. Any woman would have made the same choice as I did. I've never seen a mother desert her child, whatever the difficulties. I've never seen a mother desert her child because he's ill and infected with some disease!

So I haven't yet been able to say:

"Tshakua, you're ill. You're HIV-positive."

I do drop a few hints to try to prevent him doing anything foolish as far as sex is concerned. That bothers me a lot.

The psychologists at the hospital will have to talk to him. Let them tell him the truth about his illness since I haven't the heart myself. And, because he probably knows everything now, I'll have to summon up my courage and try to find the right moment to end my silence.

It's probably true that I ought have made myself speak at the very beginning. No doubt the problem is all my fault. But when he was babbling, "Mummy, Mummy," I couldn't upset him by saying, "No, I'm not your mother."

It never even occurred to me to think, "All these lies are going to cause problems later – I ought to make everything clear now." He was my son, and I didn't think about the future. The future didn't exist. He was my little Tshakua and always would be – my little Tshakua, who was going to grow up in my care and under my eye.

That was the choice I made then, and it's still my only choice now. I've proved it every time I've said to a husband:

"You don't love my son? All right – there's the door."

I think it was quite natural; it was my duty. Any mother who'd put her husband before her child would be a true mother no longer. And now, after having chosen for years to be a mother first and foremost, am I supposed to be able to do the opposite, and tell the one I've loved the most out of all my children that I'm not his mother at all? But if he isn't my son, who is he? What would I have sacrificed all those years of my youth for?

Now that he's older it would be even worse. How could I add to his sorrows? He'll have to help me! Why doesn't he ask questions? He'll find out by himself anyway. When they're older, children feel more independent. Perhaps one day he'll say to me:

"And anyhow you're not my mother!"

I'm waiting for that day.

But when it comes and I hear those words I'll be in despair.

But as far as his illness is concerned the matter's urgent: he must be told about it now, this year. I realize this because he's starting to notice girls, and to say things like:

"Mum. the girls made fun of me because of my lace-up shoes..."

But then he's sure to ask how he contracted the illness, and that's what terrifies me. How am I to bring his mother back into the story? He doesn't even remember her. When she came he called her Auntie; I was the one he called Mummy. He slept in my room; it was I who changed his nappies, gave him his meals, did everything for him. He knew her only as his Auntie; ever since he's been able to think and recognize people, I've been his only mother. I'll never try to get that idea out of his head unless he mentions it first. Ever since he was capable of loving a mother I've occupied a mother's place. Am I supposed to tear myself out of his heart at the same time as he hears about his illness? I couldn't do it. When he hears those most terrible words – HIV-positive, AIDS – is he to be left all alone, without a mother to console and cheer him? What mother could do such a thing to her child?

Let the social workers and the rest, the psychologists, do it if they like.

I'm on very good terms with my friends and fellow-countrymen now I don't need anything any more. When you're in real trouble you haven't got any friends: I've learned that from experience. Not that I blame anybody. Friends can't really help you. They can give you a hand from time to time, as Sylvie did when I hadn't got a roof over my head. But you can't expect any more than that. She made that plain herself:

"If you were on your own," she said, "I'd let you stay on. But with the children – no, it's out of the question."

If I was rejected by everyone it was because of the children; and the one who caused me the most difficulties was Tshakua. If I was rejected both by my friends and by our community as a whole, it was because I had the children. And to keep my children with me I've fought against the authorities; for them I've come close to sleeping in the street, I have slept on the floor. For them I've stolen, accepted all kinds of humiliation, accepted everything.

Everyone thought I was obstinate, stupid, mad. They wondered how I managed, how much I earned to be able to steer my course all on my own. The social workers expected me to give in. They'd even given me the phone number of the duty officer at the Social Services so that someone could come and get the children at any hour of the day or night. But I never used that number. No one wanted to know about my troubles. It was my own look-out if I thought I could do without the services provided for people in my situation. That made me all the more stubborn. And I won.

My friends and I get on very well now.

When the town hall gave me this flat, the only person I told was Sylvie. Of course, after she turned me and the children out of her place, things were a bit strained between us for a while. But as none of it would have happened if it hadn't been for the children. I didn't resent it for long and she was still my best friend.

"Sylvie, thank God! I've found a flat!"

I didn't feel like telling the others: they'd rejected and made fun of me, and I had another idea up my sleeve for them. One Saturday, as soon as I was settled in, I tidied up the flat and got a buffet ready, and some drinks. No one except Sylvie knew this was where I was living now. On the Sunday we went to church as usual.

At a certain point in our church service the congregation is asked if anyone wants to bear witness.

That day I stepped forward and witnessed;

"Glory to God," I said. "Thanks to Him my troubles are over. I couldn't find anywhere to live. I didn't have enough money to pay a council house rent, but I sent in an application anyway, and after three months the town hall gave me a four-roomed flat! I think it's God's doing, and so I want to bear witness that He has given me a lovely big house! I'm very, very pleased, and that's why I stand before you to witness to God's greatness and to His love for me. And I invite the whole community to come and see my new house. I've got some nice things ready for us all to share."

Outside the church, after the service was over, they all came up to congratulate me.

"How on earth did you do it?"

"How did you manage it?"

I was happy to tell them.

They all came back with me and we made up. I don't bear them any grudge. I'm not angry with them – Adrienne, Emilie, and the men who left me. We're great friends now. I chose how I was going to live my life, and I don't blame anybody else. I was the one who made the men leave. They went because I wanted to keep my son.

They were within their rights. It's not for me to judge them. The Bible says, judge not, that ye be not judged. But if I had judged Kasongo when he left me and the children alone without a roof over our heads, I'd have thought, "He's a swine and I never want to set eyes on him again." Still, when he asked if he could have Tshakua for the holidays I was pleased. And even though he brought him back again and I was upset, I didn't blame him. I just explained:

"Tshakua's only a child, and if he sulked it was because he found you living with someone who isn't his mother."

The same with that West Indian woman. I wanted her to know how I felt, but I don't bear her a grudge. It's just fate. Everything is ordained before we're born – there's no such thing as chance. Everyone does what he has to do. Whatever he does is natural, and he can't be blamed for it. As for me, I know how I lived back in the village, and now I'm in Europe and I'm somebody. What's become of the people who stayed back home, and what sort of progress have they made, I don't know. But God prepared my way for me before I was born.

When the minister came here from Rwanda he shared out responsibilities among the congregation. He appointed deacons and deaconesses. I'm a deaconess now. I started taking the church seriously when I fell ill, back home.

Even before I went back I'd often had attacks, in all sorts of places. Once the fire brigade had to come and collect me in the metro. My first attack happened at work: I was cleaning the toilets and tried to pick up my bucket and found I couldn't move. I yelled! The man who was working with me was vacuuming at the time and didn't hear me at first. I went on shouting and finally he came. He tried to help me, but I still couldn't straighten up. So he went and fetched the concierge and they rang for an ambulance, and I was taken to hospital. The doctors did all sorts of tests and sent me from one department to another, one hospital after another – Créteil, Beaujon, and so on. But they couldn't find anything wrong. I was swallowing doses of medicine from morning till night. The only explanation they could find was that I'd had too many worries... One doctor said it was a nervous breakdown; another said it might be the start of some mental illness and wanted me to see a psychiatrist; a third had another version – they all had different points of view. But I thought to myself, "It's grief, because my sister's just died."

I went and consulted some Muslim holy men – I wasn't a good Christian yet. I'd already been to see a holy man when my sister was taken to hospital. He said someone had cast a spell on her at the airport. And now I thought, "That spell has passed on to me!" It seemed to me the same power that had harmed my sister had transferred its attention to me now she was dead. And the holy man said he was sure I was right.

During all this time I was getting no better. The doctors did what they could. I was taking tranquillizers all the time, and minerals – all sorts of things. When my mother was ill and I went to see her, I took a huge supply of medicine on to the plane with me.

And I always kept my handbag with me wherever I went: there was a note in it from the doctor, saying what needed to be done if I had an attack. The effect of the medicine I was taking lasted about three hours, and then I started shivering. It was as if the medicine was a drug and I was having withdrawal symptoms. Sometimes I just couldn't move. I was like a statue – I couldn't even speak. I still don't know what was wrong with me.

Back home, in the capital, I went to church and saw the minister. He listened to what I said and then asked:

"How much medicine are you taking?"

I showed him all the things I'd brought with me. He poured paraffin over them and set them alight. When they were all burned up he said:

"Do you believe that God, who gave you life and breath, can cure you?"

"Yes."

"Very well. Stand up. You're cured. You don't need any medicine – it wasn't medicine that cured you. Now you are in the power of God."

From that day on I haven't felt faint and I haven't taken any more medicine. On that day I saw the power of God. And I decided to read the Bible and find out about His miracles and how He guided the children of Israel. And I started to be a practising Christian. I had gone to church before, but I hadn't taken religion seriously. But on that day back home I really saw God's miracle.

When I was young I was a Catholic, because I'd gone to Catholic schools. I don't condemn any religion. Everyone's free to choose his own. But I've noticed that the Catholics always say the same prayers. It's "Hail, Mary, full of grace" today, and tomorrow it will be the same. But when I joined the Pentecostal Church I discovered something else. Now I can speak with God myself. He sees me and listens to me. And I've found a new way to talk with Him. "What am I, God, before Thee?" I talk to him, tell him all that happens to me. And I always get an answer! And so I'm a sister, I'm free, and I obey the commandments I've read about in the Bible. And I tell God everything. I know I'm a sinner, but I won't confess to a man. Another human being can't pardon me. I speak directly to God, and ask Him to have mercy on me.

At home I say my prayers every night before I go to bed – not long prayers, but always something. And every morning when I wake up I give thanks to God, and in particular I thank him for giving me life and breath. This is the most important moment for me, because not everyone's had the blessings I've been given. Then I pray that His peace be with me, and ask Him to come with me wherever I go. That's all. And I say everything inside my head, without speaking aloud: that's how it is when you speak from the heart.

I still have to lie to everybody, which I hate, but I know all my troubles and anxieties and problems are necessary for my son's sake. If I could overcome my reluctance and say he has this illness, he's the one who'd suffer. For example, when he stays away from school it's because of his illness, But I can't one who'd suffer. For example, when he stays away from school it's because of his illness, But I can't answer the teacher's questions truthfully. She may be the teacher, but she's also a woman like any other, and I know what people are like. And the other children mustn't find out anything, either. And the same with the people I know, the friends I take him to see. Everywhere he goes, God knows I have no choice but to lie.

I can't even bring myself to speak freely to Sylvie. Perhaps one day, when she's asked me round to her place and we're chatting together, I may tell her everything. I don't know. She and I talk about everything, AIDS included. But I can't tell her the truth. I just can't.

I don't want my son to be rejected, you see. I want him to lead a normal, carefree life. I want him to have friends, to enjoy himself, to be safe in a happy world. I want him to have the same life as other people. My darling.

To protect the anonymity so important to
Thérèse some of the names of people and places
have been changed.

AFTERWORD I

The Professor of Medicine in charge of Tshakua's treatment.

In my hospital we remember the story of this boy and his mother as if it happened only yesterday. We were naturally struck by the fact that while the mother died of AIDS, the child somehow managed to survive. For hers was one of the first cases of the disease to be identified: the earliest diagnoses date from October 1982. One or two unusual cases had already cropped up where, looking back now, we know the patients in question were suffering from AIDS. But we were unaware of this at the time.

The mother arrived in Paris early in April 1983, without any papers and without any money. Three days later she had an epileptic seizure and was referred to us by another hospital for an abscess on the brain. At first we couldn't diagnose what was really wrong with her, because in those days we'd never come across toxoplasmosis. In the end, however, her illness was identified as AIDS and treatment was begun. Unfortunately the disease ran its full course and in November 1985 the patient died within forty-eight hours of a sudden attack of septicaemia. Hers was one of the longest-surviving cases of cerebral toxoplasmosis.

She was from an African country which for personal reasons she'd left in haste, bringing her youngest child with her. Something now had to be done about the boy, both from the social and from the medical point of view, though as to the latter he didn't yet present any major problems. He was just over six months old when he arrived in France, and HIV-positive, though we were unaware of that at the time: the AIDS virus was not identified until February or March 1983, and no serological tests were yet available. As a matter of fact we couldn't confirm that the child's blood contained antibodies until over a year later: before that, though we might suspect that he was infected, we couldn't be sure. He was one of the earliest certain cases of transmission from mother to foetus, and we still didn't know the extent to which the disease was passed on from parent to child.

He's at present one of the longest-surviving cases. There aren't many of them anyhow: children infected in this way either have a rapidly developing form of the disease and die within a year or two, or if, as in his case, the illness takes a more lingering form, their condition deteriorates faster than his has done... There has so far been no major worsening in his condition.

So the baby's early problems were chiefly social: where was he to go? His mother was seriously ill, and here all alone except for her son. Her friend, Madame Muamini, had difficulties of her own at that time and couldn't take the child in. So to begin with, from 1984 to 1985, he was looked after in a crèche run by the Department of Health and Social Services. The people there had objected at first because they didn't really know if he was infected or not, nor what kind of risk there might be to the other children. In a series of long telephone conversations we insisted that they must take charge of him: where else was there for him to go? The Department of Health and Social Services was a public service, we said, and it was the duty of the state to look after any homeless child in his circumstances! But he genuinely did present the crèche with a novel problem, and the doctor there was in a dilemma: it was his duty to accept the child, but he also had to protect the others: the familiar conflict between the welfare of the individual and interests of society.

In the end the Social Services did keep the boy, though until September or October 1986 we used to take him back into the hospital occasionally and then return him to the crèche. By that time Madame Muamini had found somewhere to live, and the Social Services handed the child over to her.

Other difficulties cropped up with the headmistress when he was sent to school, a year after his mother died. In those days the press and public opinion were obsessed with the question of whether HIV-positive children should be allowed to go to ordinary schools, and controversy raged about the risks of infection. I can still remember my phone conversations with that headmistress. "But what's the matter with the child?" she asked. "I've got nothing to say," I answered, "except that he can and must go to school like any other child, and that's all there is to it." The family who'd adopted him was plagued with questions too, but finally the matter was settled and the little boy duly went to school.

His medical progress is monitored all the time, but there have been no serious adverse developments so far and his height and weight are normal. He does have some problems at school because he can hardly read or write. But of course there've been complicating factors. And he's a nice lad; if his behaviour's sometimes a bit rowdy it's because he's very robust.

Unfortunately, as we can tell from our experience with patients slightly older than he is, other problems may lie just ahead. He's now eleven and a half, and will soon start asking questions: why must he keep taking medicine, why does he have to come to the hospital? Whether such questions arise sooner or later will depend on how fast he develops mentally, how curious he is and what things he happens to see or hear. But arise they will. And the problem of sex is bound to crop up in the next two or three years. Things will get very complicated.

But it isn't up to me to solve such problems: that task will fall to Mme Muamini, though we can help her cope with them. We're already in touch with Professor B., a child psychiatrist, on the

AFTERWORD I

problems confronting such children and those who have taken the place of their parents. Professor B. will see the boy and his family and advise his adoptive mother on what and what not to tell him, and how and when to talk to him. For he can't be left without answers to all the questions he's bound to ask as he approaches adolescence.

As to the future, it's hard to know what to say. Quite possibly, one day, a deterioration may set in, an infection occur, or some other adverse development. But at the age of eleven he is one of the oldest surviving cases of mother-foetus infection, and he has been brought up in conditions as satisfactory as circumstances allowed. Once the early upsets were over, life became more stable for him, and as he was one of the first children to present society with the HIV problem, his story has served as a prototype, helping to get other such children accepted by schools and by the authorities in general.

Thanks to his adoptive family, his home and social background have been as good as could possibly have been hoped. I should like to pay tribute here to his adoptive mother, and to thank her for all she has done to help this little boy. Any credit there may be in this story belongs entirely to her. And, believe me, it hasn't been easy.

AFTERWORD II

A British Perspective

In the last decade, since the first cases of HIV infection and AIDS were reported, it has been recognised as a significant childhood health problem in many parts of the world. In the UK, as in other parts of Europe, the numbers of children infected by mother to child transmission are still relatively small but are increasing yearly, particularly in urban areas such as London and Paris.

We have come a long way in understanding the course of the disease in children born with HIV. Research studies in Europe have told us that only 1 in 5 to 1 in 6 children born to positive mothers will themselves be infected. And we now know that although about one fifth to a quarter of these will become quite seriously ill in the first year of life, many children are living with the disease through childhood and starting to enter adolescence.

Increasingly we know more about how to prevent transmission from mother to child – for example by avoidance of breast-feeding or by use of the anti-HIV medicine, AZT, in pregnancy.

In the UK, over 300 children born to HIV infected mothers are known to be infected themselves with HIV, the majority living in London. As in Paris, major children's hospitals have responded by setting up centres of expertise and an effective way of managing all the medical, psychological and social aspects of the disease in a whole family has been found in the development of family-based clinics. The idea is that team members working in these multi-disciplinary clinics can offer a wide range of expertise and care through different stages of the illness, as well as liaising with local services.

Over the last three years, paediatricians caring for children with HIV throughout Europe have come together to share their expertise, undertaking studies about the transmission, natural history and treatment of the virus. One of the organisations co-ordinating such studies is the Paediatric European Network for Treatment of AIDS (PENTA).

Dr Diana Gibb
Honorary Consultant Paediatrician/
  Senior Lecturer in Epidemiology
The Institute of Child Health,
  Great Ormond Street Hospital
June 1995

June 1995
Tshakua's illness entered the active phase...

The Astonishing True Story of Lord Nelson's Coffin

Told in the coffin's own words,
recounted here by Julie Hall

*For Gill
with best wishes
Julie Hall*

ISBN 978-1-85580-067-0

First published in 2018 by QMSL on behalf of The Nelson Society
www.nelson-society.com

Copyright © 2018 Julie Hall. All rights reserved.

Cover and illustrations by Robert Amos
rob.amosculturalworker@gmail.com

A CIP record for this book is available from the British Library.

Typeset in 12/15pt Monotype Garamond by BluemoonPrint, Bristol.

Printed and bound in the United Kingdom by Quay Digital,
Portishead BS20 7AN.

THE NELSON SOCIETY

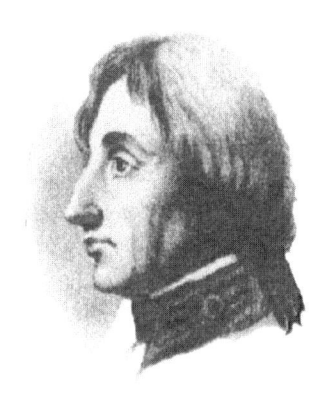

The Nelson Society is a registered charity whose object is to advance public education in the life and achievements of Admiral Lord Nelson and other related topics.

The Society aims to support appropriate good causes relevant to Nelson and his world with advice, consultancy and grants to research and conservation projects. There are no headquarters to maintain as we are managed by a committee of volunteers elected from the membership.

Membership is open to anyone who is interested in the life and times of Nelson, his navy and his "band of brothers". Members are sent our Journal The Nelson Dispatch free of charge and are able to participate in our lively and varied social programme. To find out how to join go to our website: www.nelson-society.com

Profits from the sale of this publication will be used to support the charity.
Registered Charity No: 296979

ACKNOWLEDGEMENTS

At the time of writing, Julie Hall was Membership Secretary of The Nelson Society. She wishes to thank the following people for their contributions to The Astonishing True Story of Lord Nelson's Coffin. Sue Miles and the staff of The Nelson Museum, Monmouth, for making their collection of Nelson-related books available for study; former TNS Chairman Louis Hodgkin for his help with ship-building knowledge and historical details; Janet Hendley for her comments on style; TNS Vice-Chairman Ray Aldis for sorting out which French Admiral actually died propped up on a chair aboard *L'Orient* at the Battle of the Nile (amongst other things); TNS President The Hon Peregrine Nelson Hood for allowing the use of the photograph at the back of the book; Susan Amos for suggesting her son as a suitable illustrator and Jeanette Ryder for being one of the first to read the story and to enthuse about its potential.

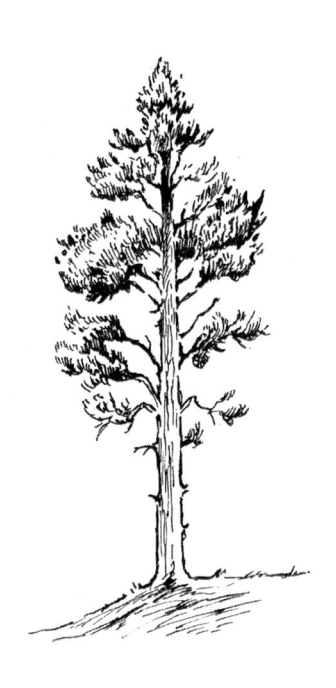

CHAPTER I

My first memory is of being dropped from a great height by my mother. It was not that she was careless or negligent, but at that moment on a chilly autumn day many, many years ago, she felt that she had done all that was required of her and so she let me go.

I felt the impact, but not too severely as I was safely tucked away with my siblings. We hit the forest floor and bounced a little way away from Mother, coming to rest in a soft and springy layer of pine needles which had accumulated over time and nicely cushioned our landing. The hob-nailed boot of a hunter caught us as its owner crept through the forest in search of a suitable animal which would be sacrificed to feed his family. We landed some way away from Mother in a more exposed location and settled down to wait for the return of the spring sunshine.

I won't trouble you with an account of the 80 or so years that followed, except to say that I grew strong and straight, proudly thrusting ever higher into the sky above my head with my girth increasing nicely. Nothing much bothered me in those days. I endured icy winters and gloried in warm summers. Small animals and birds occasionally made their homes in my branches, but on the whole, I was left in peace to grow.

One day, the habitual tranquillity of the forest was interrupted by men's voices calling to one another close by. Then, a sound which became familiar to me from time to time over the next two decades or so invaded my consciousness. It was a harsh sound which heralded my future existence: the sound of a crosscut saw. The first cut is the deepest as the saying goes and this was quickly endured. The lumberjacks who came to harvest me were experienced in their work and once they had begun sawing, I was soon parted from the roots which had sought and provided nourishment during my years of growth. Once my side branches had been removed, the journey began. The place which I had called home for so many years was soon left behind, with nothing but a rotting stump to act as a grave marker and hint at my passing.

CHAPTER II

Hustle and bustle. Men are rushing here and there. Time is money and, in this port, there is plenty of money. Agents from Britain, agents from France and Spain, agents from Holland, their purpose is the same. Europe is a politically unstable continent and many of its governments are anxious to build ships to defend their coasts from possible aggressors, whilst others pursue ambitious expansion of their territories. These countries have become adept at securing the best materials for the construction of their growing navies and the means to do this are not always "above board". There is much talk of piracy: some of the cargoes which have lately been destined for France or for the Dutch shipyards have mysteriously disappeared en route. Ships need masts and my country of birth is now the go-to supplier of the necessary trees. This is what I glean from the conversations around me.

I am resting on top of a pile of other harvested tree trunks which have been just been inspected. We are known as "hand masts" because our circumferences are measured in palm widths. I am proud to say that I have been marked as a "K" grade, which means I am a future top-quality mast. Some of my neighbours have been awarded a "B" or even a "BB" which makes them less valuable than me. I believe I am destined to serve an important role, but at this stage in my story, I have no idea how ultimately famous I will become.

After a great deal of waiting around on a damp quay, I am finally hoisted aboard the specially built merchantman which will transport me to France. It is a long and perilous journey, not just because of the risk of being stolen by an enemy along the way, but because it is a long voyage from the Baltic Sea to the Mediterranean and bad weather, poor seamanship and ill-fortune in a hundred other ways, may prevent our arrival in Toulon.

The captain of the merchantman on which I occupy quite a lot of deck-space, is a wily old sea dog and has experienced many similar trips. He is the veteran of an act of piracy by a British ship (conveniently showing quite a different country's flag) and is determined not to be caught in such a way twice. His sole mission is to sail as fast as is practicable to Toulon, ignoring entreaties from other vessels pretending to be in difficulty as had previously been the case and fleeing as far and as fast as possible from any other ships spotted from the crow's nest look-out aloft, in order to avoid trouble. Apart from any other considerations, there will be a weighty bounty for safe delivery of this cargo, some of which he may choose to share with his hard-working crew.

The voyage seems interminable. The ship is tossed about day after day in high winds which whip up salty waves to break, time and again over my prone length. Lashed together with coarse ropes, the soon-to-be masts pitch and roll with the weather. Brave sailors going about their dangerous business occasionally stagger into us and bark their shins when the storms are particularly vicious, causing them to swear and curse. We will all be glad to be ashore once more.

CHAPTER III

Our arrival at the French port of Toulon is greeted with much enthusiasm, not just by the weary crew, but by the men on the quay who rapidly release the stacks of tree trunks from the deck and hoist them with some care onto dry land. It quickly becomes clear from the sights and sounds around me that we have arrived in a place where fighting ships are built. Ships nearing completion are being rigged by an army of craftsmen under the watchful eyes of their masters.

We are separated out into lengths and grades and gradually dispersed, dragged away by sweating and straining horses to a quieter area of the shipyard where there is a mast pond. So this is my destiny: to become a mast on a fighting ship. Having already come so far, I hope that my duty lies with worthy and famous commanders: I will serve gallant captains and victorious admirals for years to come. Of course, at this moment I could have no notion of what form my service would take, nor how long my connection with one particular heroic seamen would continue into the future.

For now, however, the pond is where we will lie quietly for some months to come, immersed in the salty water. We will be pickled by the brine and so become much less likely to twist, split or rot once stepped aboard our ships. I am used to being patient; I will dream of future glory, dimly aware of the glaring hot sun above, but of little else.

* * *

A rude awakening. The time has come for the next stage in my existence. Brought out once more into the open air, each tree trunk is inspected and floated to the ramp of the mast house. Next, we are propped length-ways on short, specially made supports to keep us off the ground and allow the flow of warm Mediterranean air to circulate around us and soothe away the dampness we acquired on the long voyage and later in the mast pond.

CHAPTER IV

The mast house is a hive of activity. It is a huge timber-framed building with a saw pit over which tree trunks are suspended to be cut by two men - one above and one below. Some of the masts-in-waiting repose suspended on old ship's "knees" which are attached to beams supporting the building. Much of the work done here must be very precise, as I learn when the master shipwright arrives with his plans and his calculations. To find the height of the main mast (that will be me) he will add together the length of the lower deck to the extreme width of my ship-to-be and divide it in half. Or at least that is what I think they said....

I had imagined standing tall aboard my ship all in one piece but that is not how strong masts are made on mighty warships. I am of course to be the sturdy base of the mast and I am to be cut into square sections, then tabled together, before they round me up with an adze. The joints will be reinforced with bolts, tightly bound with rope and then the blacksmiths will be called in to make iron bands which will be heated up. Once they are fitted around me and then cooled down again making them shrink, they will make me as strong as can be and ready to be fitted or stepped into the hulk of the ship. Or at least, that is what I think they said....

I am starting to realise that all this technical detail is, on the need-to-know basis, not something I should worry about. Once I am ready for use, I will be hoisted by masting crane mounted up over the deck by two lifting blocks and manoeuvred until I am over the mast opening. They will drop me into place until my foot engages the mortice in the stepping keelson. I will be kept in place by stays and shrouds made from tarred rope. Or at least, that is what I think they said....

Time passes. You know by now that I don't mind feeling the seasons change and biding my time; it is the very nature of a tree. From landing in Toulon, until the day when all is ready for the launch of my ship, many months have passed. All manner of workmen have had a hand in creating me, the main mast, although a man named Jacques-Noël Sané seems to be taking all the credit for the ship as a whole.

Finally, on 20th July in the year 1791, we are launched. Such excitement. You can only guess at my emotions when we are named *Le Dauphin Royal* in honour of the French Royal family and I learn that we are to be the flag-ship of the French fleet in the Mediterranean. Compared with many of the other vessels produced by this shipyard, we are huge, dwarfing others nearby. We will be fitted with 118 cannon and over 1,100 men will live, work and perhaps fight, on board.

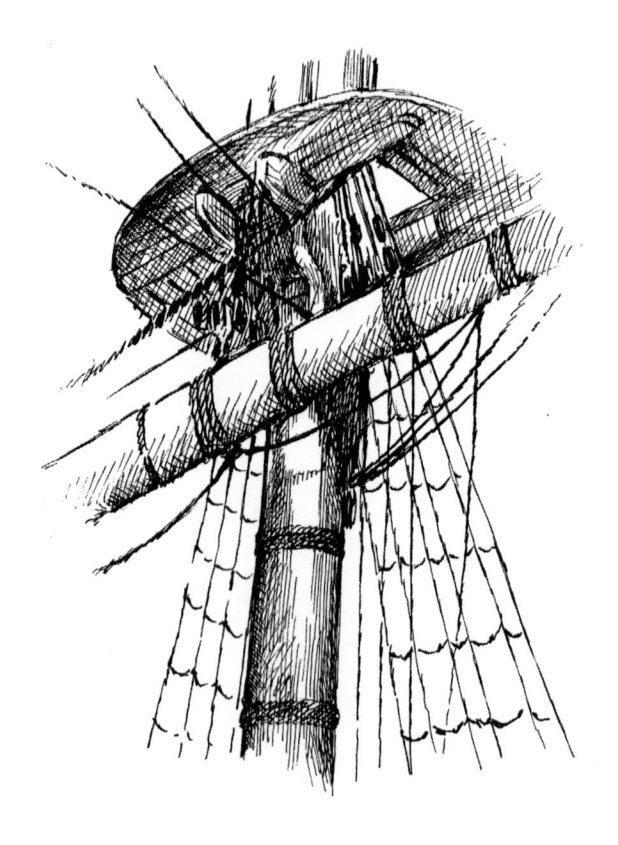

CHAPTER V

Politics! Just as I had become used to my splendid birth name and royal connections, everything changed. The France of Louis XVI which had needed me for many reasons, most of them linked to war with our British neighbours, became the France of revolution and republic. Being called *Le Dauphin Royal* (Royal Prince) became an embarrassment almost overnight and after thinking (though not very hard in my opinion) about how to honour my new masters, my ship was re-named *Sans-Culotte* after the poor but brave men and women of the revolution. I could not help but ponder the actual words: "Sans" - without; "culottes" - breeches, or short trousers. I hear many things and I came to understand that this term was used to mean people who wore working trousers instead of the impractical silk breeches of their masters. Still, it took me some time to get used to the idea. I was fitted with a new figurehead depicting a revolutionary, designed, no doubt, to put fear into the heart of any enemy getting close enough to see this fearsome, muscular giant. Mind you, I was never sure about the addition of the floppy red rosetted hat as it seemed at odds with the classical heroic pose and classical symbols he was supplied with, including his Herculean club and *"faces"* or bound rods meant to represent Roman justice.

We have sailed in and out of the port of Toulon many, many times. My crew is very nervous, I can tell, as we can all hear the cannon fire from the shore beyond the town. The whispers are that the British, Spanish and a variety of Italians have ganged up on revolutionary France and are engaged against them on land. Toulon, a Royalist town, is being besieged having invited British protection.

It is getting close to Christmas (no Christmases any more for the atheist revolutionaries of course, God save them) in the year 1793 or for them, the newly named year II. The captain of *Sans-Culotte* has a bad feeling, he says to his second in command. He orders us to set sail and there are soon men scrambling aloft into my height to begin the process of unfurling the sails which will catch the wind. Later, the sky in the direction of Toulon is aglow. The British, it seems have decided to evacuate, but before they leave, their last action is to destroy the arsenal and set fire to the eight ships still anchored in the harbour. Thanking God aloud for saving them is now forbidden, so the men aboard *Sans-Culotte* merely think it.

It is a well-known fact that most deaths aboard fighting ships occur not in battle, but through disease, malnutrition or more commonly accidents, often from falling down from somewhere high up onto the unforgiving deck below, or falling down into somewhere wet - The Sea. Luckily for the majority of my crew today, the only casualty was caused by missed footing high in my rigging, as a young sailor struggled with a tricky knot, overbalanced and screamed piercingly as he plunged my length to his death on the deck below. The fact that he landed head-first was a likely a blessing as it spared him a lingering and painful demise. Had we still been in port, it could have been so much worse as the British could well have destroyed us.

CHAPTER VI

All is not well! It is plain that with the change from Royalist to Republican commanders (many of the Royalists having completely and literally lost their heads, I learn), much expertise has been lost. There is an idea amongst the officers in charge of the gunners, that they should attack the enemy - by which I mostly mean the British as we are now allies of Spain - by trying to hit their rigging. As a supporter of rigging (yes, I know, but I enjoy just a little light humour even on the darkest of subjects) I can understand why this would disable an enemy ship. However, as we are soon to find out, the British plan is to aim for the biggest target possible - the ship itself.

In the meantime, here we are in 1795, or year IV as we must call it. We have Rear Admiral Martin aboard and he is commanding a fleet of fifteen ships which has been charged with re-conquering Corsica. Oh, the ignominy! We can't take part in the action on 14th March, which is *Pâquerette* or Daisy Day by the revolutionary calendar (I can't resist telling you that tomorrow is *Thon* or Tuna Day and the one after that *Pissenlit* or Dandelion Day) because we have somehow acquired a damaged tiller. We return to Toulon having missed the action, during which two other vessels having been lost.

* * *

It is May 1795/ Year IV. For reasons I don't quite understand we are to be renamed once more and from now on, you must call my ship *L'Orient*. Apart from this, little changes: Rear Admiral Pierre Martin continues to hoist his flag on board. My crew is ill-trained and ill-disciplined, apparently though, and Martin has to be ruthless in putting down a possible mutiny amongst the men. He is helped by a government official called Niou who tells the men "to wash their crime in the blood of the enemies of the French Republic". Ringleaders are rounded up and the punishment for insurrection is death. I will not go into detail, but I bear witness to much suffering of the culprits and stony silence from those fortunate enough not to be held accountable.

July. We are now at the head of a fleet, recently reinforced, of seventeen ships. The sun beats down on us as we are discovered by a British flying squadron off Cap Corse. The Captain of this squadron will, in time, be utterly linked with my own destiny. It is later that I learn his name is Horatio Nelson.

It becomes clear that there is little to be gained at this moment from a full-scale battle against the British, whose own commander is Vice Admiral Hotham. We seek a safe anchorage off the Isles of Hyères, but one of our number, the ship bringing up the rear is caught and having already surrendered, catches fire during the action. Some 300 of the crew of *Alcide,* for that is her name, are killed when she blows up. I have now witnessed the terrible fate of a vessel when her stores of powder cannot be protected and she explodes, showering the sea around her with torn and twisted wood, metal and men. I can only hope that this is not the future which awaits me.

* * *

Much of the next three years or so goes by in a blur. We are baked by the sun, buffeted by the wind and often playing cat and mouse with the British, although it seems that we now have the upper hand. One day, I am curious as to why my ship is being so thoroughly cleaned and spruced up (a very apt expression for a tree with my pedigree!) All is tidy, clean, stowed and scrubbed when a short, but obviously charismatic man is brought aboard amidst much pomp and ceremony. Ah, so this is the leader to whom the whole of France now looks: General Napoleon Bonaparte.

The quarter deck of *L'Orient* becomes the meeting place where Bonaparte discusses his plans to attack Malta and Egypt, thus causing severe disruption to British trade, amongst other things. Tactics are discussed; toasts are drunk and speeches given and warmly received. At last, it would appear, I am to be a vital part of a grand vision. *L'Orient* is to be the flag ship leading a massive expedition of 280 ships, thousands of men and guns. We will be commanded by Captain Luc de Casabianca, himself under the orders of (newly promoted by Bonaparte) Vice Admiral Brueys and assisted by Chief of Staff Honoré Ganteaume. What an honour to have so many distinguished men aboard….

* * *

…But wait! There is too much aboard; I can feel it. Too many officers, too many men and too many guns. When we finally try to leave Toulon where we have been so overloaded, disaster is only just averted as we touch the bottom. There is a massive, collective intake of breath as we finally struggle to get underway, but behind their hands, the sailors, always deeply superstitious, whisper that this incident is the direst of ill-omens.

CHAPTER VII

The crew may have been concerned by the grounding incident due to the weight of our burdens, but their commanders appeared to have no such scruples. After all, the ship has been well made with all possible modern features and continues to be used to ferry the chiefs of the army, including General Bonaparte, wherever necessary.

The objective of capturing and pillaging Malta was achieved: indeed, we avoided the British blockade and I learn from the boastful talk of the men aboard, took the island with relative ease. Now we are to take troops to Egypt so that Bonaparte can continue his seemingly unstoppable conquering of valuable territories. Oh dear! This, I am afraid, is where everything finally began to come to grief.

You will be relieved to learn that we are now using the old calendar again, so I can say that the next and most fateful day, will be known for ever as 1st August 1798. We are too big to enter the harbour at Alexandria as much of the dock has been destroyed in fighting. We therefore find ourselves at anchor away from the coast, seventh from the ship in the van and six from the rear, so *L'Orient* is at the centre of the fleet and our formation is deemed by Admiral Brueys to be correct if we need to defend ourselves from an unlikely British attack.

I don't think that Horatio Nelson, commanding the enemy fleet is aware of the fact that he is unlikely to attack! Nelson is aboard his flagship *Vanguard,* which boasts a mere 74 guns compared with our 118, when he happens upon the French ships at anchor. Still, there are fewer British ships and we are feeling sure of ourselves after recent successes. Little do we know all of our advantages in numbers will count for little or nothing in the ensuing battle.

A British ship is almost alongside us. I don't believe this was intended by its captain as it led to the ship - the *Bellerophon* - being all but destroyed. We begin firing our cannon at the shortest of ranges and the immediate effect of the first massive round of roaring and blinding light, is the death or injury of some 70 members of the enemy crew. It is hard to describe the chaos and deafening noise of a sea battle. There is so much smoke from the guns that things become murky and blurred. There is a cacophony of noise: apart from the dreadful noise of the cannon, there is the exploding and splintering of timber and the horrible wrenching of rigging being ripped apart and thrown down. Injured men scream and officers bellow orders trying to be heard over the din and it all goes on for hours on end.

Worryingly, I am beginning to feel very hot. If you are wooden, this is an extremely unhappy state of affairs. No doubt this is partly due to the firing of the cannons and the pounding of the enemy cannon balls smashing into us. All around me men are scurrying between the wounded and dead and splintered wood from the deck and my own spar. They shout that there is a terrible problem: the pumps which are used to keep the areas around the powder stores dowsed and therefore safe from catching fire, have been damaged by enemy guns. Our victory over the *Bellerophon* has been short-lived. Although she has been dismasted and horribly damaged so that her only option was to float away from the action, her place has been taken by not one, not two, but three other British ships. *Swiftsure, Alexander* and *Leander* are taking it in turns to attack us. As we are the largest and most prestigious ship of the fleet, this is no surprise.

Hotter and hotter. This may not end well for us. Our courageous gunners are now having to man both broadsides simultaneously. Speaking of courage, Admiral Brueys is displaying unbelievable valour. He is still in overall command, even though he has lost both his legs to a cannon ball. He has ordered the surgeon to tie tourniquets around the bloody stumps of his limbs and he is propped atop a chair on the deck near my ever-increasingly hot length, when another roundshot puts him out of his misery by removing his battered head.

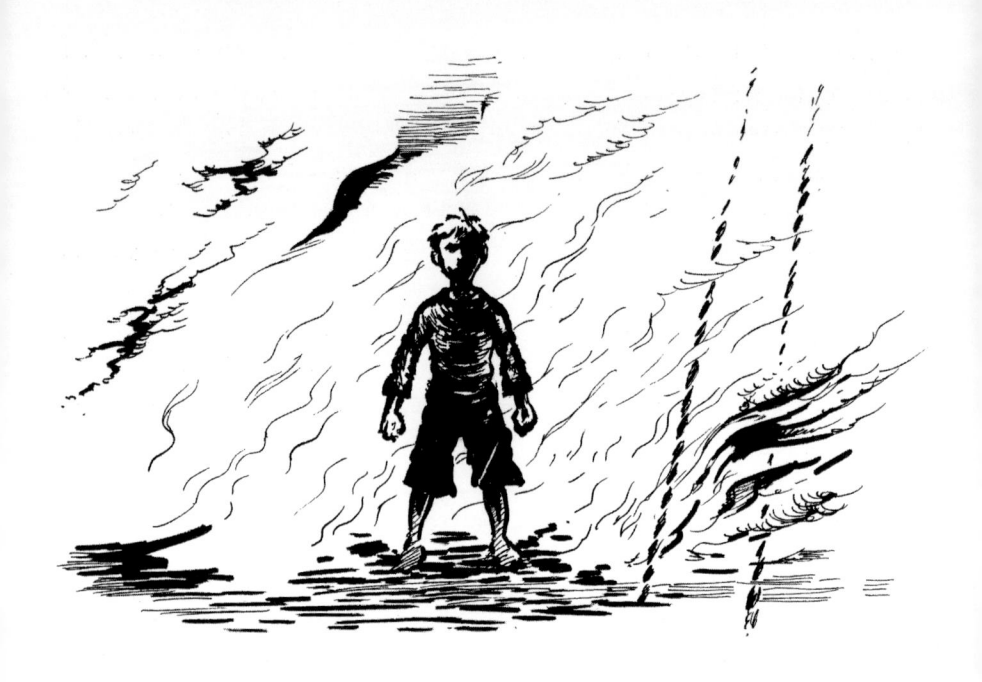

Also aboard, Rear Admiral Ganteaume is assembling as many of the officers as he can find and demanding their advice, shouting to be heard over the screaming wounded and the roaring of the cannon and all the while dodging flying debris and flaming sails and rigging as it falls. If the crew had been able to flood the magazines, there might have been a chance to save the ship, but this is proving impossible under the sustained and deliberate bombardment of *Swiftsure* and *Leander*. I hear the words: "Sauve qui peut" ("Save yourselves if you can") being repeated all around. Below decks, they do not know of this decision and amazingly, keep firing, right up until the destruction of their ship.

Brueys may have been in charge of the fleet, but *L'Orient* is commanded by Captain Luc de Casabianca. Also aboard is his young son. Legend has it that the gallant captain cannot bear to abandon his vessel, even when it becomes apparent that all will very soon be lost, and cannot allow his son to do this either, thus setting a poor example to the rest of the men. Many years in the future, this brave, but ultimately futile act will be written about in a poem called Casabianca entitled "The boy stood on the burning deck" by a poet called Felicia Hemans. It is my deck. Little does the child know that his father is lying unconscious below decks and so could not even change his mind and his order not to abandon ship if he wanted to. It has grown dark. Still the battle rages and still the heat is building around me.

If a poem was written about the tragic human aspect of the day which came to be known as the Battle of the Nile or Aboukir many, many artists have tried to capture the final moments of my brave host *L'Orient*. And what final moments they proved to be. We must not forget that she is a mammoth ship, massively manned and equipped. When the two powder magazines finally blow up almost simultaneously, there is an explosion which surely would have rivalled any volcanic eruption. So huge is the noise that there is a pause in the battle. I know relatively little of this as I am launched like a rocket from my place on the ship and shot upwards into the smoky sky, so high that it seemed hours before I come back down and land with an almighty splash in the sea. Survivors cling to me. Debris, some of it human body parts, keeps falling all around me like macabre rain. All manner of destruction, so hard to remember, never mind recount, continues to be wrought all around. Apparently, a cannon weighing 2 tons will later be found 400 yards away. Men who had miraculously jumped clear and had not been blown to pieces, were rescued by boats from both sides.

And I drift helplessly amongst the carnage, expecting this to be the end of my role in history, thinking I would become fuel for some beach-comber or other…

…But as I am still here to tell my story, it is clear to you that was not to be my destiny….

CHAPTER VIII

Gradually, survivors are dragged from the water by boats lowered from the least damaged of the remaining ships. The heat of the explosion had caused the pitch aboard the neighbouring vessels to melt and run in streams down their sides and there were many other consequences including massive holes in the hull and sails hanging in tattered rags from broken spars. Some of the human flotsam, amongst which is Lieutenant Berthelot of *L'Orient*, had saved himself by jumping from the blazing ship naked, (his clothes had been smouldering) with only his battered cocked hat as proof that he was an officer. No one will ever know for sure how many lives were lost or forever altered that day.

A day, perhaps two, after the explosion-to-end-all-explosions had blown *L'Orient* to smithereens, the salvageable marine wreckage is picked up, mainly by those looking for a trophy to remind them of the battle and with luck, show to their children and grandchildren. The victorious Nelson himself acquires the main top gallant mast head, which he will keep as a private trophy. One of his captains, Benjamin Hallowell, finds and fishes out of the water more substantial parts of the mast floating around aimlessly. I know this, because it is what is left of me!

Although most of what is recovered is kept by the British as a memento, Captain Hallowell has quite another idea about what to do with me. After I have been stored for some time amongst all manner of items in the hold of *Swiftsure*, I am finally to begin my new role and with it, my rise to fame. Under Hallowell's supervision, I am released from the hold and carried back up above by a couple of sweating and swearing sailors to be handed over to the ship's carpenter.

As you know, I have experienced being cut and shaped before. The carpenter measures and saws, saws and nails and finally I am ready to be inspected by Captain Hallowell. When he sets eyes on me, he nods and congratulates the carpenter for a job well done. A cheeky young midshipman called John Lee occasionally climbs into me as a joke once I had taken my new shape, until it was suggested that I could be nailed shut, which soon put a stop to this sport. I am put to one side in the workshop, leaning against the wall, until the time will be right for me to be handed over to my new owner.

Later, time means little to me really, so it could have been hours, days or weeks, the Captain returns to the carpenter's workshop and looks over my new form of a six-foot long shallow box. After some thought, he sits down at the carpenter's workbench and having asked for a pen, ink and some paper, he writes the following note which is then pasted onto me:

"I do hereby certify that every part of this coffin is made of the wood and iron of *L'Orient*, most of which was picked up by His Majesty's ship under my command in the Bay of Aboukir. - *Swiftsure* May 23rd 1799 - BEN HALLOWELL."

A coffin! Well, I am content to be useful and since my career in the French navy is clearly now over, at least I am to be given a new role, important no doubt to someone once their worldly life is over. Captain Hallowell is writing again and this time he reads the words aloud as he writes:

To "The Right Hon. Lord Nelson K.B.
My Lord
Herewith I send you a coffin made of part of *L'Orient*'s main mast, that when you are tired of this life you may be buried in one of your own trophies but may that period be far distant, is the sincere wish of your obedient and much obliged servant. Ben Hallowell."

A coffin for Lord Nelson… now that is an un-looked for honour. I have heard his name spoken so often, both aboard *L'Orient* (Napoleon Bonaparte was definitely not enamoured and neither were his officers) and now aboard

Swiftsure, that I know he is a famous naval personage. Aboard *Swiftsure* his name is uttered with quite a different tone: the British sailors love him and consider him to be a great tactician and brave commander, but one who is also conscious of the welfare of the men serving under him. It is something of a relief therefore, that Captain Hallowell writes of a distant time when I will be needed. As usual, I will wait patiently.

With some difficulty, I am carried up to the open air and rested briefly on the deck. Captain Hallowell has summoned a young midshipman to him. He instructs the poor lad, a fourteen-year-old youth whose name I learn is Henry Masterman Marshall, to accompany me in the captain's barge now being lowered down to the water, to deliver me to my new owner: Lord Nelson himself. The word amongst the crew is that he is in something of a black mood just now. There is mention of a lady (Emma? Frances?) who may be responsible for his depression, although I have no idea why.

It is an awkward journey between ships; a coffin is an ungainly object and not easily transported. I can feel the tension in young Henry as he considers the task he has been given. He is not sure if he has drawn the shortest possible straw if Lord Nelson is offended by the gift, or the best possible advertisement for himself as a trusted member of Hallowell's crew if the coffin is well-received.

We arrive alongside *Vanguard* and arrangements are made for me to be hoisted from the barge onto the deck using halyards of the main yard and a certain amount of muscularity from the waiting sailors.

Now for the moment of truth. Henry is breathing hard and perspiring freely in his uniform under the hot sun. His Lordship has arrived and is standing next to me, a slight figure with one empty sleeve which is pinned to the front of his coat and a face showing livid battle scars. Perhaps his need of me will come sooner rather than later after all. He spends some time looking me over and is presented with, and reads, Hallowell's note. There is silence. Then the great man himself bursts into laughter, revealing a mouth sparsely furnished with teeth. He pats young Henry on the shoulder with his remaining hand and bids him send his compliments to Captain Hallowell and thank him for such a thoughtful gift. Henry is dispatched back to *Swiftsure* mightily relieved.

I am allowed pride of place for some time on the quarterdeck. When Lord Nelson spots some of his officers staring at me in astonishment, he calls sternly: "You may look at it gentlemen as long as you please but depend upon it, none of you shall have it." He then has two crewmen remove me from the quarterdeck and place me in the great cabin where I stand behind his dining chair like a waiter ready to serve him. Well! This is indeed a new honour.

For the next few weeks I stand proudly behind His Lordship's chair. I hear every word which is spoken by Nelson and his officers. He is the first commander to defeat Napoleon in a battle and there is much talk of what will happen next in the war. The Admiral seems unconcerned by my presence, but I notice some of his officers now eyeing me uneasily. Perhaps they sense their own mortality, or maybe that of their beloved chief. It is possible that Lord Nelson himself grows tired of such a symbol of what is to come, especially on the days when he is plagued by a headache or the stump of his arm aches and reminds him of how vulnerable he is. Whatever the reason, eventually the order is given to put me carefully in the hold.

After what seems like a short while though, I am once again in the bright sunlight as in June 1799, I am taken, along with other precious objects, aboard the next home of my owner: his new flagship *Foudroyant*.

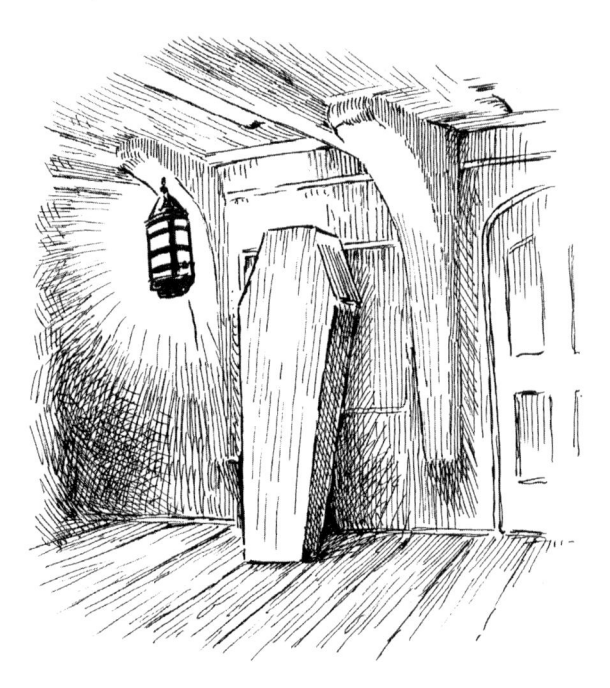

CHAPTER IX

I suppose I should be happy to be missing all the action. After all, my days as a vital part of one of the greatest warships ever built for the French navy did not end well ("C'est le moins qu'on puisse dire" or if you are not a French speaker like me, "That's the least we can say".) Newly recruited to the British cause, I must be glad that I am not yet needed to fulfil my destiny. However, in the dank darkness of Foudroyant's hold, all I can do is try to make sense of the voices I hear around and above me. I have gleaned that we are stationed near Naples, where those Frenchmen, never lacking ambition, have occupied the city.

No, wait. My new owner has once again intervened (how the French must hate him!) and in aiding the King of Naples to overcome the invaders, he has been created Duke of Brontë in Sicily. Is there no end to His Lordship's heroic deeds? There is fortunately nothing for me to do for the 9 months I am ashore in Palermo, which is to say, he is still very much alive. Lord Nelson is twice absent, once to Minorca and once Malta, but I hear little of this.

Finally, we are recalled "home", wherever exactly that is, and so a rather long and arduous journey begins. Brought out once again into the warm sunshine, there is little time to shrug off the dampness of the cellar where I have been lying, before we undertake a short sea voyage, after which I am manhandled onto the back of a wagon at a place called Leghorn.

I perch amongst trunks full of clothes, boots, hats and books, all of us covered with a rough sheet and secured with a rope to stop us from jumping about too much over the rutted and pot-holed roads which will be our hosts for many days. Off the cart once more and aboard another ship (terrible weather and a truly foul-smelling and horribly wet hold) until we arrive in Trieste. Next, we trundle on to Vienna. I may have neglected to mention that the wagon transporting me is one of three carrying baggage. There are also fourteen coaches and perhaps a hundred horses with us. This is necessary because our party contains The Queen of Naples who is on her way to Vienna. We stay in Vienna for more than 5 weeks and whilst I remain in a store room, His Lordship is wined and dined as the hero we all know he is. What I know, I hear from the grumbling attendants who are to accompany us "home".

    Each night when we have been on the road and when the bumping and jolting finally stops, my wagon is detached from the horses who are eagerly led away to their rest and food in stables. From time to time, I am party to a visit from His Lordship when he leaves his lodging for some air after dinner. He is often accompanied by a lady whose voice I come to recognise. There is a great deal of whispering and sometimes long silences, although I can sense they are still nearby: of course, I am covered up and cannot see what is happening. Some of the conversations concern a man called Sir William who, it would appear, is the lady's husband. I know little of relationships of course, but these two seem very close and it is slightly confusing that His Lordship's most frequently uttered phrase which I can make out is "Oh, My Darling Emma".

    I lose track of the places we visit and the time we spend travelling. It has been decided, I gather, that in order to avoid even more dangerous and uncomfortable travel by road, we will take to gondolas and sail down the river Elbe. This we do until we reach Hamburg where His Lordship had expected to find a navy frigate to take us "home". Hearing him nearby talk through what sounds like gritted teeth, I understand that he has had to hire a mail boat called **King George** to get us to England. Even now, we are to endure another five-day voyage, which as it November, is a stormy affair. I fancy that I even feel the boat go aground at one point on a sandbank before we finally arrive in England, at Great Yarmouth to be precise. I cannot help but remember the grounding which occurred on our departure from Toulon aboard **L'Orient** and the ensuing bad luck prophesied by her crew...

    I am sure that there are some who enjoy travel, but frankly, I have seen a lot of action since leaving the glade in my mother's stately forest and I am no longer a stripling. I suppose I will come to call "home" wherever His Lordship is when he finally ceases his rootless wandering. Is it wrong to hope that one day soon, I may just be allowed to rest quietly and dream of my native forest, whilst of course carrying out my most important duty of keeping safe the mortal remains of Admiral Lord Nelson?

CHAPTER X

London. After more jolting and bumping along in the company of Lord Nelson's luggage, we arrive at the place where I am to spend around the next five years with not much to do but wait. I am to be kept in storage at the premises of Messrs Marsh, Page and Creed of Norfolk Street, The Strand who look after other belongings for my owner and act as his agent. During this period, I have no contact with the outside world and therefore have no news of the deeds of my master, although I must suppose that he is away doing his duty (something of which he was often heard to talk in my presence and which he took extremely seriously) to his country and king.

Then one day in the early autumn of 1805, I am disturbed by a candle-lit visit by Mr Marsh in the company of Lord Nelson. He has come to discuss a number of issues concerning his estate. He has the air of a man putting things in order in the knowledge that he may not be much longer for the world. I don't believe that this really has any immediate bearing on my future, until a heavy metal candle-stick is placed on my lid and I hear him instruct Marsh to have my history engraved upon me. "I feel that I may have need of Hallowell's gift soon now", said His Lordship as his agent retrieved the candle and the door to my store-room was once more securely locked. I hear my visitors' retreating footsteps down the tiled corridor and wonder what His Lordship can mean.

CHAPTER XI

No doubt you have more knowledge than me of how His Lordship met his end. I was not there in *Victory* Nelson's Flagship at the Battle of Trafalgar, on 21st October 1805, when a French sniper in the tops aboard the *Redoutable* aimed his musket at two officers walking the middle of the quarterdeck and succeeded in hitting the shorter one with the stars on his coat. I didn't hear this officer say to the other: "They have done for me at last, Hardy," to which this gentleman, his friend, replied: "I hope not", and to which His Lordship answered: "Yes, my backbone is shot through."

    I did not witness Nelson's agony-filled last moments when he had been taken below and seen by the surgeon William Beatty, who could do nothing for him. The Reverend Doctor Scott did his best to comfort the Admiral as his life ebbed away four hours later. I heard tell of the last visit of Captain Hardy to Nelson's side, as this had a bearing on my future part in Nelson's own story. His Lordship stated adamantly that his body should not be thrown overboard, to which of course Hardy agreed, all the while telling his dear friend and intrepid commander, of the great victory which had been won over their enemies. In his darkest hour, as well as his famous triumph, His Lordship was thinking of Captain Hallowell's gift which was lying in readiness back in England; he was thinking of me.

    Amongst Horatio Nelson's last audible words was a phrase he often repeated: "Thank God I have done my duty", which so poignantly echoed the memorable telegraphic signal he had ordered be made to the fleet before the battle: "England expects every man to do his duty."

***

You probably know that in order for His Lordship's wish for a funeral in England to be fulfilled, a means has had to be found for his body to be preserved during the voyage home. His hair was cut off and most of his clothes (except for a shirt) removed. He was then put into a leaguer - or large cask - which was filled with brandy. The brandy was often drawn off and replaced with a fresh supply, which was mixed with spirit of wine after a stop in Gibraltar. I understand that this worked so well, that when, on 11th December the body was taken from the cask it appeared perfectly preserved.

It will soon be time for me to become a permanent home to Lord Nelson. The door to the store room in London where I have patiently waited is opened and I am carried out into wet and windy cobbled street by two porters, who slide me carefully onto the back of a wagon. This time, there is no need to share the space with other baggage and in fact, I am handled with a reverence which I have not before experienced as I am covered outside with black silk and padded inside with white satin. This does not mean that the next part of the journey is particularly comfortable though: the roads are bumpy, rutted and muddy and the poor horses pulling the wagon often struggle in the wintry conditions and are whipped frequently by our driver on the way to Chatham Dockyard.

I have quite lost count of the number of times I have been on and off a seagoing vessel. From the day I left my native country in the north as a raw tree trunk, to my proud days as part of the main mast on France's largest and most important ship *L'Orient*, then aboard *Swiftsure* having been rescued from the sea, before being taken to meet His Lordship on *Vanguard*, I have travelled far and wide. Couple this with the journey back to England in 1800, there can rarely have been a pine tree as well-travelled as me. So, as I am once again transferred from the land to the sea and my appointment with my destiny aboard *Victory*, I take it all in my stride.

Strong hands grasp me as I am swung aboard and I then find myself taken to His Lordship's cabin. In the after-part of this, there already stands a wooden coffin. I can't say whether it is at this moment or before, that I am lined with swathes of white silk. With much ceremony, the other coffin is opened. It seems somewhat indelicate to describe what happens next, but soon, the mortal remains of Admiral Horatio Nelson are once more dressed. A night-cap is placed on his head as if to send him off to a good night's sleep and he is placed reverently inside me and covered with a shroud. I am then placed in a leaden coffin which is soldered up and like a Russian Doll, we are placed inside another wooden casket.

***

As the hero who has saved the nation from invasion by Napoleon and has made England the master of the seas, Lord Nelson will be given a state funeral the likes of which have not been seen before and are unlikely to be witnessed again. There are days of public lying in state at Greenwich and a private attendance for the Prince of Wales and other privileged persons before the general public is allowed to file past me. Some 15,000 do this, but many more are turned away. Of course, I can only hear all of this going on dimly.

On 8th January 1806, we leave Greenwich and take to the River Thames, which, as we ride very close to it, feels as choppy as any water I have been on in my naval career. My precious cargo would have been mightily pleased to see the number of barges in the river procession and even happier to know of the quality of the royal and otherwise noble or notable passengers carried in them.

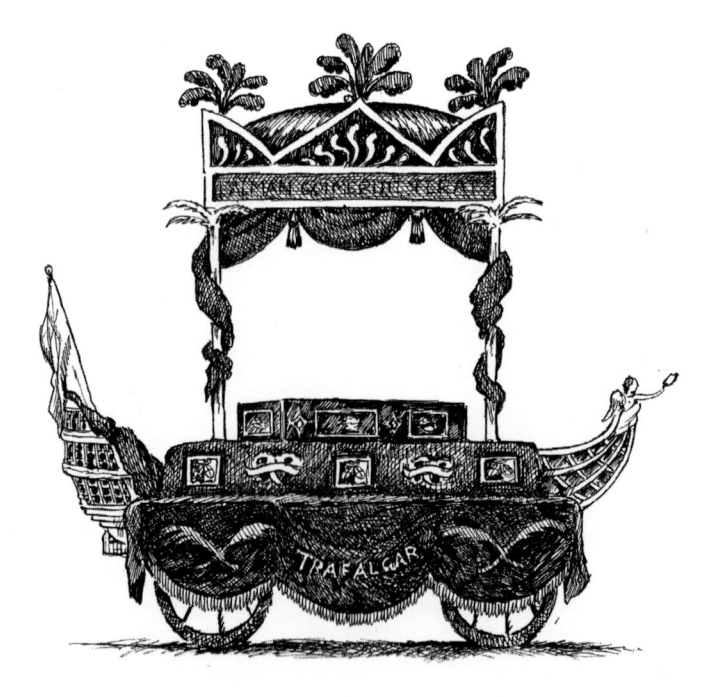

The sound of the great guns firing at minute intervals from the wharf and being answered by the gunboats in the procession, recalls to me the battle in which my career as a mast ended and my destiny as a coffin began. We are brought ashore at Whitehall Stairs with some difficulty, due to the frankly awful weather and the state of the tide. This caused the late and much-lamented Lord Nelson to pitch and toss in his shroud, I can report. There is even a portentous clap of thunder.

After staying the night at The Admiralty, the following day seems interminable. The noise of the crowds as we jolt along in our no-doubt spectacular funeral car is at times deafening. The wonder of the on-lookers penetrated the darkness as they pointed and described our carriage, adorned with a scaled down model prow and figurehead of the flagship *Victory,* the whole towered over by a magnificent canopy topped-off with black ostrich plumes and the Viscount's coronet of His Lordship. Eventually we come to a complete halt and we are lifted (by twelve sailors due to the weight of three coffins in one) from the funeral carriage and carried into St Paul's Cathedral where hundreds of people have been waiting for hours. There is singing from a 100-strong choir and solemn organ music aplenty. The service itself is long and emotionally charged.

Hours later - it seems - the funeral service finally ends with the words: "His body is buried in peace but his name liveth evermore." You will understand the sketchiness of the details here. Lord Nelson is now safely encased in layers of wood, metal, marble and my own protective cocoon and we are thus distant from the reality of what is happening outside.

***

For more than 200 years under the golden orb of the dome of St Paul's Cathedral, Lord Nelson's tomb has been visited by friends (and old enemies), relatives, admirers and those seeking inspiration from proximity to the fallen hero. We hear many, many languages spoken by our visitors, who usually adopt a respectful and hushed attitude as they draw near, sometimes depositing wreaths, posies and other tributes. And so, here my story ends, although of course, my duty of keeping the body of Britain's greatest naval commander safe for all eternity does not…

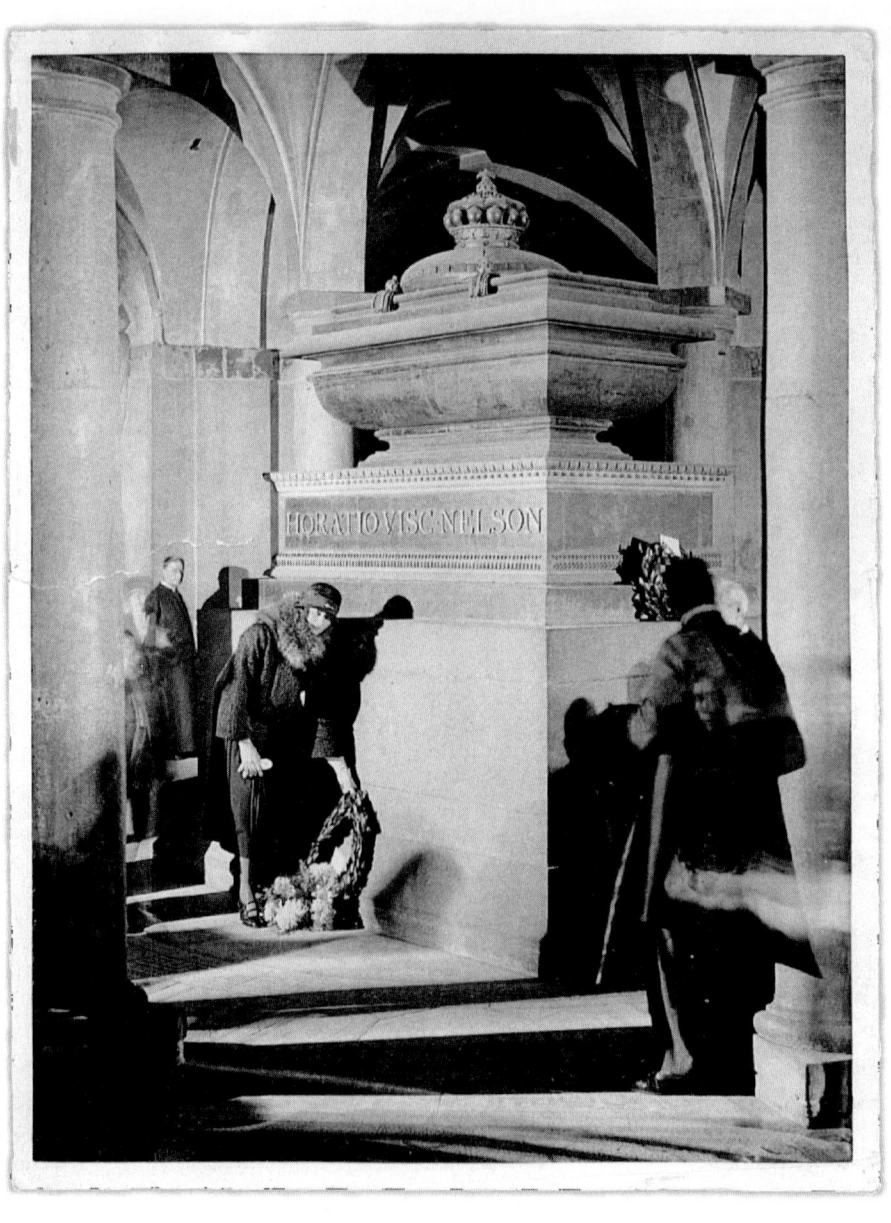

*The photograph is from a family diary of Sir Alec Nelson Hood,
Duke of Bronte - it shows Trafalgar Day in 1922 and the Duchess of Sutherland
on behalf of the Navy League placing a wreath on Nelson's tomb.*